IMMUNOLOGY AND IMMUNE SYSTEM DISORDERS

IMMUNITY AND IMMUNOTHERAPY OF HUMAN FUNGAL INFECTIONS

Immunology and Immune System Disorders

Additional books in this series can be found on Nova's website under the Series tab.

Additional E-books in this series can be found on Nova's website under the E-books tab.

IMMUNOLOGY AND IMMUNE SYSTEM DISORDERS

IMMUNITY AND IMMUNOTHERAPY OF HUMAN FUNGAL INFECTIONS

MAWIEH HAMAD
AND
KHALED ABU-ELTEEN

Nova Science Publishers, Inc.
New York

LIBRARY OF CONGRESS CATALOGING-IN-PUBLICATION DATA
Hamad, Mawieh.
Immunity and Immunotherapy of Human Fungal Infections / authors, Mawieh Hamad, Khaled Abu-Elteen.
p. ; cm.
Includes bibliographical references and index.
ISBN 978-1-61728-976-7 (hardcover)
1. Mycoses--Immunotherapy. I. Abu-Elteen, Khaled. II. Title.
[DNLM: 1. Mycoses--immunology. 2. Mycoses--therapy. 3. Immunotherapy.
WC 450]
RC117.H356 2010
616.9'69061--dc22
2010028487

Published by Nova Science Publishers, Inc. ✢ New York

CONTENTS

PREFACE

Immunity and immunotherapy of human fungal infections is an up-to-date in-depth assessment of the current status of immune-based antifungal preventive and therapeutic interventions. This book consists of integrative chapters that deal with the subject from different angles. Also discussed herein is an updated review of medically important fungi, the diseases they cause, morbidity and mortality trends that associate with them, conventional antifungal chemotherapy, and non-immune-based (actual and/or potential) unconventional treatments. The intended audiences of this book include, but are not limited to, students, researchers, and practitioners in the general fields of immunology, mycology, dermatology, and allergy.

Chapter 1

HUMAN FUNGAL INFECTIONS: BASIC BIOLOGY AND EPIDEMIOLOGY

In the last two decades, risk-factors for , incidence of, and mortality due to invasive fungal infections (IFIs) have all been on the rise. The ever-increasing number of hosts with compromised immunity as a result of underlying diseases (cancer, AIDS, diabetes, etc.) or immunosuppressive therapy (cancer patients and transplant recipients) is largely to blame for this open-ended vicious cycle [1, 2].

Although *Candida albicans*, *Aspergillus fumigatus*, and *Cryptococcus neoformans* are the most common causes of IFIs [3], a recent increase in the incidence of infections caused by *Candida* and *Aspergillus* species other than *C. albicans* and *A. fumigatus,* opportunistic yeast-like fungi (*Trichosporon* spp., *Rhodotorula* spp., and *Geotrichum capitatum* or *Blastoschizomyces capitatus*), zygomycetes, hyaline molds (*Fusarium*, *Acremonium*, *Scedosporium*, *Paecilomyces*, and *Trichoderma* spp), and dematiaceous fungi has been noticed (table 1.1).

Throughout this chapter, and while reading subsequent chapters, it is probably useful to be reminded that host-parasite relationships are determined, to a large extent, by a delicate balance between fungal pathogenicity and the competence of host immunity. The disturbance of body defenses has increased greatly with the use of antibiotics, immunosuppressive drugs, hyperalimentation fluids, polyethylene catheters, pressure monitoring devices, heroin abuse, organ transplantation, abdominal surgery, and prosthetic cardiac valves [2-7].

Table 1.1. Spectrum of opportunistic fungal pathogens

Candida spp.	*C. albicans* *C. glabrata* *C. gulliermondii* *C. kefyr* *C. krusei* *C. lusitaniae* *C. rugosa* *C. parapsilosis* *C. tropicalis*	Other yeasts Zygomycetes	*Cryptococcus neoformans* *Trichosporon spp* *Rhodotorula spp.* *Geotrichum capitatum* *Blastoschizomyces spp.* *Malaseezia spp.* *Saccharomyces spp.* *Absidia spp.* *Cunninghamella spp.* *Mucor spp.*
Aspergillus spp.	*A. fumigatus* *A. niger* *A. flavus* *A. terreus*	Dematiaceous molds	*Rhizopus spp.* *Rhizomucor spp.* *Alternaria spp.* *Bipolaris spp.*
Other hyaline Molds	*Scedosporium spp.* *Fusarium spp* *Acremonium spp.* *Paecilomyces spp* *Trichoderm spp.* *Scopulariopsis spp.*		*Curvularia spp.* *Cladophialophora spp.* *Exophiala spp.* *Phialophora spp.*

YEASTS AND YEAST-LIKE FUNGI

Candida

Candida albicans is commonly found in the gastrointestinal tract, oral cavity, and genital area as a harmless commensal. As well as being harmless commensals, *C. albicans*, and other *Candida* spp. are opportunistic pathogens that cause a range of different infections [3, 6]. Based on recent studies in healthy individuals, asymptomatic oral carriage of *Candida* spp. is estimated to occur in 24-70% of children and adults, with a reduced frequency in babies less than 1 year of age. Of isolates identified, the majority are *C. albicans* (38-76% in adults and children). Again, the frequency of *C. albicans* differs across different age groups, with a far greater proportion of isolates identified as *C. albicans* in young babies and the elderly. Higher oral carriage rates are found in HIV positive patients [8] and diabetics [9]. Asymptomatic vaginal carriage of *Candida* spp. occurs in 21-32% of healthy women, with *C. albicans* representing 20-98% of identified isolates [6, 10-12]. Beigi *et al* [13] have reported that within a group of women repeatedly screened over 12 months,

30% were never colonized, 70% were colonized on at least 1 occasion, and 4% were persistently colonized. Higher rates of vaginal carriage have been found in pregnant women, women colonized by *Lactobacillus* spp [13, 14], type I diabetics [15], and post-antibiotic treatment [12]. Table 1.2 summarizes the various predisposing factors to candidiasis along with specific examples of diseases associated with high incidence of *Candida* infection.

Table 1.2. Factors predisposing to *Candida* infections

Factors	Observations	Examples
Neutrophils defect	Myeloperoxidase deficiency results in abnormally small number of neutrophils in circulating blood	Acute leukemia, chemotherapy, irradiation
T- lymphocytes		AIDS, Hodgkin's disease, chemotherapy
Reticuloendothelial system (RES)	Congenital or surgery-related defective RES impairs clearance of infectious particles from blood; this is due to	Defective spleen function, splenectomy
Chemotherapy and Radiotherapy	Treatments that alter the composition of the endogenous microbial flora or suppress immunity	Immunosuppressants, antineoplastics, antibiotics, corticosteroids
Interrupted integument	Membrane trauma, burns, local occlusions or tissues macerations	Finger or bone marrow punctures, gastrointestinal (GI) ulcers, catheters, IV needles, wearing dentures
Surgical procedures	Introduction of mechanical devices and prostheses into vessels or tissues	Heart valve replacements, respiratory assistance, endoscopy, renal transplants, heart surgery, GI or gynecological surgery, blood transfusion
Physiological factors	Debilitating diseases and disorders (idiopathic, congenital, acquired), diviations from normal physiological status	Microbial infections, endocrine dysfunction, defective cell-mediated immunity (CMI), pregnancy, infancy
Nutritional factors	Feeding habits that create an environment conducive to the development of mucosal candidiasis	Carbohydrate-rich diets, vitamin deficiency

Superficial mucosal infections: Superficial mucosal lesions (thrush) commonly occur in the oral and vaginal cavities in both immunocompetent and immunocompromised hosts. Oral candidiasis is a common problem seen in infants, the elderly, and cancer patients, particularly those with hematologic malignancies receiving chemotherapy or head/neck radiation. It is characterized by white growths on mucous membranes of the oral cavity with underlying red areas following yeast growth scrapping [16]. The majority of isolates associated with oral candidiasis are identified as *C. albicans* (63-84%)[17]. Risk factors associated with oral candidiasis include xerostomia (dry mouth) and denture wear [17, 18], poorly controlled diabetes mellitus [9], and immunosuppression (table 1.3). The frequency of oral candidiasis, but not oral carriage of *Candida* spp. [19], is higher in HIV positive patients with decreased $CD4^{+}$ T cell counts [8].

Vulvovaginal candidiasis (VC) represents a real health problem to women of childbearing age worldwide where the genitourinary tract commensal *C. albicans* is encountered in >80% of cases [6, 10, 11]. The occurrence of VC and recurrent vulvovaginal candidiasis (RVVC) has been attributed to compromised immunity and increased levels of estrogen in the reproductive tract milieu (table 1.3) [20]. Symptoms of VC include itching, burning, soreness, and abnormal vaginal discharge. *C. glabrata* has emerged as an important and potentially resistant opportunistic fungal pathogen of VC [3]. It has been demonstrated that among the *Candida* spp., *C. glabrata* alone has increased in incidence as a cause of VC in Jordan since 1994 [21]. In fact, the rising trend of *C. glabrata* as a common cause of VC that is becoming increasingly resistant to fluconazole chemotherapy seems to be a worldwide phenomenon [2, 3, 22].

Bloodstream *Candida* infections: *Candida* bloodstream infections (BSIs) (candidemia) represent the fourth leading cause of nosocomial BSIs in the United States [3,6, 23]. The annual incidence of *Candida* associated BSIs in the USA and Europe is in the range of 6-23/100,000 [24, 25], and 2.5-11/100,000 individuals [29] respectively. In recent years, there has been a gradual increase in the incidence of BSIs [27-29] with more than 17 different *Candida* spp. identified as etiologic agents. Approximately 95% of all *Candida* BSIs are caused by four *Candida* spp., namely: *C. albicans, C. glabrata, C. parapsilosis,* and *C. tropicalis* [30,31], With some variations among different patient groups, *C. albicans* remains responsible for the majority of infections (42-100%) while the rest are caused by 12-14 different spp. including *C. krusei, C. lusitaniae, C. guilliermondii, C. dubliniensis*, and *C. rugosa* among others [3,6,25,26,32-35]. For example, the ratio of *C.*

albicans to non-*albicans Candida* in patients with hematological malignancies is about ½ that in patients with solid tumors [26, 34]. Although *C. albicans* continues to be the most common spp. in both Europe and the United States, epidemiologic data regarding other *Candida* spp. suggests different patterns of distribution in different regions of the world.

Table 1.3. Specific factors predisposing to neonatal, oral, and vaginal candidiasis

Factor	Type		
	Neonatal	*Oral*	*Vaginal*
Physiologic factors	Prematurity, mother-placental insufficiency, hyperbilirubinemia, pathogenic *E. coli* in the stool, genetic disorders, prolonged pre-delivery labor	Severe blood diseases (leukemia, leukopenia, aplastic anemia), malignant and chronic diseases (carcinoma, kidney disease, chronic lung disease), endocrine disorders (diabetes).	Anemia, diabetes, malignancy, pregnancy, hormonal disturbances
Interrupted integument	Birth trauma, catheters	Burns, oral trauma, dentures	
Nutritional factors	Malnutrition, breast and bottle feeding	Malabsorption	Malnutrition
Chemotherapy and radiotherapy	Antibiotic and steroid therapy (taken by mother of infant after birth) effect (psychophamaceuticals) radiation therapy	Broad spectrum antibiotics, corticosteroids, irradiation, or drugs with xerostomic side effects	Antibiotic therapy, oral contraceptives
Surgical procedures	Resuscitative procedure intubations (especially transplantation and heart surgery), tooth extraction	Parenteral nutrition, convalescence after operations	
Other factors	Unsterile delivery, male sex, unhygienic environment, low birth weight, thumb and dummy sucking, immunological factors	Poor oral hygiene, oral leukoplakia, immunological factors	Humidity and warmth, tight–fitting clothing, immunological factors

In that, whereas *C. parapsilosis* is the second most common *Candida* spp in Southern Europe, *C. glabrata* is the second most common one in France,

Germany, and England [30, 36]. *C. parapsilosis* occurs with high frequency in premature neonates and in patients with vascular catheters [36, 37]. Although *C. glabrata* infections are rare in infants and children, they occur more frequently in the elderly [3, 25, 30, 38]. *C. tropicalis* plays an important role as a cause of invasive disease in patients with hematological malignancy [3]. Overall, non-*albicans Candida* spp. are becoming increasingly responsible for a greater number of BSIs [24, 25]. This is mainly due to the increased prescription and use of fluconazole as well as the emergence of *C. glabrata* and *C. krusei* in countries like the USA [3, 38, 39]. Interestingly, the frequency of *C. glabrata*-causing BSIs has decreased in Europe (from 12.3% to 8.8%) and in Latin America from 10.2% to 4.7% [40].

In the majority of cases, those who develop candidemia are intensive care unit (ICU) patients and patients recuperating from invasive surgery. Other patient groups at risk of candidemia are cancer patients (solid tumor and hematological malignancy types), premature babies (<1kg birth weight), and those on steroid therapy [16]. In critically ill patients, several risk factors may be present in, or apply to, the same patient [41, 42]. For example, one study has reported that up to 14% of screened central venous catheter (CVC) tips were positive for different bacterial and fungal microorganisms with *C. albicans* being second to coagulase-negative *Staphylococcus* spp. [41].

Cryptococcus

The strong association between cryptococcal infections and immunodeficiency and/or immunosuppression is best exemplified by the fact that cryptococcosis ranks as the second most common cause of opportunistic fungal infections in AIDS patients. The incidence of infections caused by the encapsulated yeast *C. neoformans* has risen markedly over the last 20 years [43]. Infections occur through inhalation of small diameter (< 10 mm) yeast-like organisms, which enter smaller respiratory passages, remain dormant for a period that is often dependent on the host reaction [43-45] to then reactivate in the lungs and lymph nodes. Clinical manifestations range from asymptomatic colonization of the respiratory tract to widespread dissemination depending on the immunostatus of the host, inoculum, and degree of isolate virulence [45]. As dissemination occurs, the central nervous system (CNS) is commonly involved. The basal meninges of the brain are preferentially affected causing thickening with subsequent invasions of deeper brain tissues [45]. In the meninges, the organism appears to be suspended in a mucoid material that is derived from the capsule.

C. neoformans is a basidomycete that normally grows as a haploid-budding saprophytic yeast. As opposite mating types exist, *C. neoformans* can undergo sexual reproduction and meiosis to produce spores. Yeasts cells are spherical to oval in shape and 5-10μm in diameter. *C. neoformans* strains manifest antigenic differences that allow them to be grouped into five different serotypes (A, B, C, and D in addition to an AD hybrid) as well as different varieties. *C. neoformans* var. *neoformans* includes serotypes D and AD while var. *grubii* includes serotype A and var. *gattii* includes serotype B and C. var *neoformans* and var. *grubii* are responsible for the majority of clinical infections in immunocompromised host while var. *gattii* causes disease primarily in immunocompetent hosts [43, 44, 46, 47]. *C. neoformans* has a number of virulence factors that enable it to survive and replicate in humans [48], especially if T cell CMI is compromised. The capsule is antiphagocytic and tends to down-regulate cellular and humoral immune responses when shed into host tissues [45. Furthermore, laccases and melanins released by the pathogen interfere with the oxidative killing activity of phagocytes [45]. Production of melanin from 1-dopa by the enzyme laccase may account for the predilection of the organism to the CNS. *C. neoformans* is both an intracellular and an extracellular pathogen; it can survive and replicate within acidic macrophage phagolysosomes [49]. A host site with abundant carbon dioxide concentration favors capsule bioformation [44]. *Cryptococcus neoformans* lives in soil and organic matter containing pigeon and bird excreta. *C. gattii*, which is found primarily in tropical and subtropical regions, has been associated with several spp. of eucalyptus trees and causes infection predominantly in immunocompetent hosts.

Cryptococcus neoformans is neurotropic, and most patients with cryptococcal meningitis suffer from defective CMI. The infection occurs most frequently in association with lymphoma, AIDS, transplantation, and corticosteroid therapy [50]. In the 1980s, cryptococcosis emerged as an important opportunistic infection occurring in 5-10% of AIDS patients in the US, Europe and Australia [43]. With the increased use of fluconazole to treat oral candidiasis and with the advent of highly active antiretroviral therapy (HAART) in the mid 1990s, the annual incidence of cryptococcosis decreased markedly in developed countries. For example, in the city of Atlanta, Georgia in the US, the incidence of cryptococcosis decreased from 66 cases/1000 patients with AIDS in 1993 to 7 cases/1000 in 2000 [51]. In a recent review of cryptococcal infections in HIV-negative patients, splenectomy was reported to be a risk-factor for infection in about 3% of cases [52]. Other groups at risk of cryptococcosis are organ transplant recipients receiving immunosuppressive therapy [36] and patients with sarcoidosis and lymphoproliferative disorders. In a cohort of 306 HIV-negative patients with cryptococcosis, the predisposing factors were steroids (28%), organ transplant (18%), chronic organ (liver, kidney, and lungs) failure (18%), malignancy (18%), and rheumatological disease (13%) [53].

Non-*neoformans* cryptococci have been generally regarded as saprophytes and rarely reported as human pathogens [54]. However, the incidence of infection due to these organisms has been gradually inching up for decades, with *C. albidus* being responsible for 80% of reported cases. Impaired CMI is an important risk factor for non-*neoformans* cryptococcal infections and prior azole prophylaxis associates with notable resistance. Interestingyl, *C. gattii* causes disease in immunocompetent people in a geographically-restricted area in Australia [2, 43]. Additionally, the occurrence of invasive *C. gattii* infections in immunocompetent humans in Vancouver Island, Canada has been reported [55].

Invasive Infections by Other Yeast-Like Fungi

The frequency of invasive mycoses due to rare and emerging opportunistic yeast-like fungi has increased significantly in the last two decades [2, 3, 56]. These organisms may occupy environmental niches, they may also be found in food and water, or constitute part of the normal human microbial flora. The list of these opportunistic yeast-like fungi is long, so the discussion will be limited to three genera that pose particular threat to humans; namely: *Trichosporon* spp., *Rhodotorula* spp., and *Geotrichum capitatum* (*Blastoschizomyces capitatus*) [2, 3, 57-59].

Trichosporon

Trichosporon is a genus of basidiomycetous yeasts that inhabit the soil and colonize human skin and the GI tract [2]. Previously, all pathogenic members of the genus *Trichosporon* were considered as a single species (*Trichosporon beigelii*); however, recent biochemical and morphologic differences within the genus have been appreciated. *T. beigelii* has now been divided into distinct species, at least 8 of which (*T. asahii, T. inkin, T.*

asteroids, T. cutaneum, T. mucoides, T. ovoides, T. pullulans, and *T. loubieri*) can cause human disease. While *T. asteroids* and *T. cutaneum* can cause superficial skin infections, *T. asahii* and *T.mucoides* tend to cause deep invasive and disseminated infections. *T. ovoides* causes white piedra of the scalp and *T. inkin* causes white piedra of the pubic hair [2, 3, 56, 60- 62]. *T. faecale* and *T.loubieri* were isolated from the skin of patients with tinea pedis [63] and from adults with polycystic kidney disease [64] respectively. *T. mycotoxinivorans* is a newly recognized human respiratory pathogen with a propensity for patients with cystic fibrosis [65]. Additionally, *T. montevideense* and *T. domesticum* have also been implicated in summer type hypersensitivity pneumonitis [66, 67]. Risk-factors for infection with these pathogens include immunosuppression, disruption of mucosal tissues, and CVCs. In one study, it was reported that 63% of 287 *Trichosporon* cases occurs in patients with underlying hematological malignancies [58]. Those at greatest risk are neutropenic cancer patients receiving cytotoxic drug therapy. Less commonly, disseminated infections have been seen in solid organ transplant (SOT) recipients, burn patients, premature babies, and AIDS patients. The overall mortality rate is high with early reports putting it at 60%-80% [56, 60]. Recent developments in the diagnosis, treatment, and prevention are likely to have lowered rates of mortality due to *Trichosporon* spp. infections.

Rhodotorula

Rhodotorula spp. are basidiomycetous, encapsulated, yeast-like fungi that belong to the family *Cryptococcaceae* and sub-family *Rhodotorulodea*. The clinical significance of this group is becoming increasingly recognizable with the continued emergence of new cases [2, 3, 68-76]. Many spp. of the genus *Rhodotorula* have been described; *R. rubra, R. glutinis, R. mucilaginosa*, and *R. minuta* have been implicated as a cause of meningitis, endocarditis, ventriculitis, peritonitis, fungemia, CVC infections and keratitis [68-76]. These yeast-like fungi are found as commensals in skin, nails, and mucous membranes [3]. Although *Rhodotorula* strains appear to be less virulent than common yeast pathogens like *Candida* and *Cryptococcus* spp., *Rhodotorula* infections can cause sepsis and other life-threatening complications especially among groups at risk (patients with CVC implants, malignancies, and so on) [2, 3]. By reviewing 88 cases of CVC-related fungemia due to *Rhodotorula* spp., it has been shown that in all but one case, an underlying disease state, mainly cancer, was present. In fact, cancer was the underlying disease in 69 of the 88 cases [76, 77]. Although fungemia caused by *Rhodotorula* is rare, it is becoming increasingly more frequent in immunocompromised and critically ill patients. *R. mucilaginosa* is the spp most frequently recovered (75%) followed by *R. glutinis* (6%). *Rhodotorula* BSIs have been successfully managed with line removal, antifungal therapy, or a combination of both [76]. Mortality rates among *Rhodotorula*-infected patients are estimated at about 15% [76].

Geotrichum Capitatum

Geotrichum capitatum, formerly *Trichosporon capitatum* or *Blastoschizomyces capitatus*, is an uncommon but frequently fatal infection in immunocompromised patients, especially those with hematological malignancies [2, 3, 58, 78, 79]. It is widely distributed in nature and may be found as part of the normal skin flora. In a retrospective multicentre Italian study, the incidence of *G. capitatum* infections among patients with acute leukemia was 0.5%, with a 55.7% crude mortality rate [58]. *G. capitatum* infections present in a manner similar to that of *Trichosporon*. They occur in neutropenic patients with breakthrough infection (36% of episodes), there is a frequent fungemia (positive blood cultures) with multi-organ (including brain) dissemination, and the mortality rate is about 60-80% [79]. Also like *Trichosporon* infections, chronic disseminated forms of *G. capitatum* infections may be seen following resolution of neutropenia.

Pathogenic Filamentous Fungi

In the past few years, major advances in health care have led to an unwelcome increase in the number of life-threatening infections due to true pathogenic and opportunistic fungi. The emergence of organisms such as *Fusarium* spp., *Histoplasma capsulatum, Coccidioides immitis* as significant pathogens has important implications for the diagnosis and management, not only because clinical presentation can mimic more common diseases like aspergillosis, but also because the organisms are usually resistant to various antifungal drugs.

Aspergillus

The genus *Aspergillus* includes approximately 175 species, but only *A. fumigatus, A. flavus, A. terreus, A. niger* and *A. nidulans* have been associated with human disease [2, 3, 80]. The conidia (spores) are easily released into the atmosphere to reach the lung alveoli [2]. Invasive aspergillosis (IA) occurs almost exclusively in immunocompromised hosts. Frequent infections have been described in patients with hematological malignancies, SOT recipients, and in patients undergoing chronic intermittent hemodialysis, where the infection was associated with *Aspergillus* spp. building (ventilation system) contamination. Over the last 10 years, *A. fumigatus* has become the most prevalent airborne fungal pathogen being responsible for approximately 90% of human infections [80-83] with a fourfold increase in IA has been observed. In 1992, IA was responsible for approximately 30% of fungal infections in patients dying of cancer, and it is estimated that IA occurs in 10-25% of all leukemia patients, in whom the mortality rate is 80-90% even when treated [83-85].

Aspergillosis is still particularly common in hematopoietic stem cell transplant (HSCT) recipient. IA is also an emerging condition in patients with other causes of immunosuppression, such as SOT, advanced AIDS and treatment with newer immunosuppressive agents such as infliximab [25, 86]. Risk factors for IA include prolonged and profound neutropenia, high-grade graft-versus-host diseases (GVHD), use of corticosteroids, or receipt of HSCT from a human leukocyte antigen (HLA)-mismatched donor [39,87,88] (table 1.4). *Aspergillus* infections have been reported in 2-26% of HSCT recipients and in 1-15% of SOT recipients. The mortality rate in transplant recipients with IA has ranged from 74-92%. An estimated 9.3-16.9% death rate in transplant recipients in the first year occurs due to IA [81]. In a study which included more than 3000 recipients, of 91 cases with IA the mortality rate was 72% [89]. Other studies have reported different rates of incidence and mortality [91, 92].

Compared to a global incidence rate of 1.4%, IA occurs in 3% of lung transplant recipients, in 2.4% heart transplant recipients [92], and in 1.5-10% in liver transplant recipients [83]. IA is associated with high rates of mortality, which has exceeded more than 50% in some reports [25, 39, 87]. Higher mortality rates were noted in HSCT patients compared SOT patients (68% vs 41%) [25], and in neutropenic patients compared with non-neutropenic patients (60% vs 89%) [93]. Aspergillosis is also becoming an emerging mycosis in the ICU. According to a recent study [94], its incidence ranged from 2.7 to 58 cases per 1000 admissions, with a rate of mortality ranging between 75-95%. Most of the patients with IA present with chronic obstructive pulmonary disease and receive high-dose corticosteroid treatment as a remedy [94]. Infections by non-*fumigatus Aspergillus* spp. are becoming increasingly common [2-5, 39, 81], especially those caused by *A. terreus* [94- 97], which has been recognized as a cause of frequently lethal infections [2, 3]. Although, in certain instances, the frequency of non-*A. fumigatus* species like *A. flavus* exceeds that of *A. fumigatus*, the exact reason(s) behind such shifts are not fully understood [98].

Common clinical syndromes associated with *A. flavus*, which produces the hepatocarcinogenic compound aflatoxin, include chronic granulomatous sinusitis, keratitis, cutaneous aspergillosis, wound infections, and osteomyelitis [2, 3, 39].

Infections caused by a recently recognized new spp. of *Aspergillus* designated as *A. lentulus* have been reported [99, 100]. Recent studies have shown the new triazoles voriconazole and posaconazole to be more effective than fluconazole at preventing IA in HSCT patients [3, 39,101].

Table 1.4. Co-morbid conditions for aspergillosis and mold infections in at-risk patients

Hematological / blood abnormalities	Organ transplants
Leukemia Myelodysplastic syndrome Stem-cell transplants Acute / chronic GVHD [a] Prolonged neutropenia / Neutrophil dysfunction Chemotherapy Fungal colonization Steroid prophylaxis Cytotoxic drugs (infliximab, alemtuzumab) Use of T-cell depleted stem cell products ($CD34^+$ cells) Diabetic ketoacidosis [b] Iron overload [b] Deferoxamine therapy [b] Skin breakdown [b]	Acute and chronic transplant rejection Steroids Renal failure / hemodialysis Treatment with tacrolimus Cytomegalovirus infections Repeated transplantation Splenectomy / splenomegaly Alemutuzumab mAb therapy Diabetic ketoacidosis [b] Iron overload [b] Deferoxamine therapy [b] Skin breakdown [b]

[a] GVHD, Graft vs host disease.

[b] Relates to zygomycosis.

FILAMENTOUS FUNGI-BEYOND *ASPERGILLUS*

Several genera of filamentous fungi (*Scedosporium* spp., *Fusarium* spp., *Paecilomyces* spp.), the dematiaceous fungi (e.g. *Alternaria* spp.), and the mucorales group (*Mucor* spp., *Rhizopus* spp., *Rhizomucor* spp., *Absidia* spp. and *Cunninghamella* spp.) are emerging as opportunistic pathogens that can cause diseases in humans [2-5, 39, 102, 103]. Infections due to these opportunistic molds are usually marked by a poor response to antifungal therapy, *in vitro* resistance to most available antifungal agents, and an overall poor outcome with excessive mortality.

Scedosporium

Within the genus *Scedosporium*, *Scedosporium apiospermum* (teleomorph, *Pseudallescheria boydii*) and *S. prolificans* are ubiquitous filamentous fungi present in soil, sewage, and polluted waters. Scedosporiosis represents a broad spectrum of clinical diseases caused by the agents of the genus *Scedosporium*. Infections caused by these organisms can infect locally, spread to surrounding tissues, or disseminate to distant organs. The spectrum of diseases caused by these fungi is broad; they range from transient colonization of the respiratory tract to saprophytic involvement of abnormal airways, allergic bronchopulmonary reaction, invasive localized disease, and at times disseminated disease. These infections include skin and soft tissue infections with extension to tendons, ligaments, and bone (mycetoma); septic arthritis; osteomyelitis; lymphocutaneous syndrome; pneumonia; endocarditis; peritonitis; chorioretinitis; and endophthalmitis. In patients suffering from near-drowning consequences, *P. boydii/S. apiospermum* should be considered in the differential diagnosis as potential causes of infection, especially if pneumonia or brain abscess ensues. The two medically important species: *S. apiospermum* and *S. prolificans* represent antifungal-resistant opportunistic pathogens. *S. apiospermum*, a well-known cause of mycetoma, may cause deep-seated infections (e.g. CNS abscesses) and disseminated infections in bone marrow transplant (BMT) recipients and other immunosuppressed neutropenic individuals resulting in a crude mortality rate of 55% [102, 104-106]. *S. prolificans* causes bone and soft tissue infections in immunocompetent hosts and deeply invasive and disseminated infections in immunocompromised patients; the crude mortality rate tis about 90% [106]. Surgical resection remains the only definitive therapy for *S. prolificans* infections [56, 102].

Fusarium

Fusarium spp. is the second most common filamentous fungus causing invasive disease in immunosuppressed patients [103]. *Fusarium* spp are fungi with hyaline, branched, septate hyphae, which are of the same character as that of *Aspergillus* spp. [2-5,103]. In addition to classical risk factors such as neutropenia, GVHD, and immunosuppression [103,107], hospital water systems have been implicated as potent modes of transmission [103, 107, 108]. The frequency of fusariosis is increased in HSCT recipients and in patients with hematological malignancies [103,107]. The clinical manifestations of fusariosis cannot be distinguished from IA, although they are more often characterized by cutaneous involvement and fungemia [109]. The typical presenting characteristics of disseminated fusariosis are positive blood cultures (in up to 75% of patients) [103,107,110] and the appearance of multiple purpuric cutaneous nodules with central necrosis [103, 107,111]. Infections caused by *Fusarium* spp. are difficult to treat and often lead to death as a result of pronounced resistance to common antifungal agents.

Acremonium

In immunocompetent individuals, *Acremonium* spp. causes foot mycetomas and/or corneal infections following penetrating injuries. Infections with *Acremonium* spp., being increasingly recognized as opportunistic pathogens, occur mostly in individuals on corticosteroid or tacrolimus therapy, splenectomy patients, and BMT recipients [2, 3]. At least 35 *Acremonium* types of adult infections have been described [112]. Fifteen cases of infection with *Acremonium* (excluding mycetoma and keratitis) have been documented in children [113]. *Acremonium strictum* is the most commonly encountered species in both children and adults. The presence of adventitious forms of *A. strictum* provides a mechanism for hematological spread and dissemination. Fungemia due to *A. strictum* infections has been reported in neutropenic patients [112].

Paecilomyces

The genus *Paecilomyces*, which includes several spp. of cosmopolitan filamentous fungi that inhabit the soil, decaying plants, and food products, is usually considered a contaminant, though it may occasionally infect humans and animals. The most common species of this genus are *P. lilacinus* and *P. variotii* [2, 3,114]. *P. lilacinus* is an emerging pathogen that causes severe human infections including oculomycosis [114]. The fungus usually shows low susceptibility to conventional antifungal drugs *in vitro* and variable susceptibility to novel triazoles. A review of the literature has identified 119 reported cases of *P. lilacinus* infection in humans between the years 1964 and 2004, which included oculomycosis (51.3%), cutaneous and subcutaneous infections (35.3%), and miscellaneous infections (13.4%). Pulmonary and cutaneous infections, soft-tissue infections, cellulitis, onychomycosis, otitis media, endocarditis, osteomyelitis and catheter-related fungemia have all been reported [114]. Peritonitis and sinusitis are the most common infections caused by *P. variotii*. Lens implantation is believed to be the most frequent predisposing factor to oculomycosis. Cutaneous and subcutaneous infections occur mainly in SOT and BMT recipients, although surgery and primary/acquired immunodeficiencies are also relevant predisposing factors. Infections in apparently immunocompetent hosts have also been reported. A case report of *P. lilacinus* infection in a liver transplant patient has been reported [115]. The 56-year-old male patient was in his 12th month post-liver transplant when he experienced a history of painful, erythematous nodules over the right knee. Several biopsies yielded a mold that was initially phenotypically identified as a *Penicillium* species. However, sequence analysis later identified the suspect pathogen as *P. lilacinus*. Surgical debridement combined with antifungal drug therapy or the correction of predisposing factors (e.g. neutropenia) is usually warranted to improve therapy outcome.

Trichoderma

Trichoderma spp., previously considered as nonpathogenic fungi, are often used by the biotechnology industry as a source of enzymes and antibiotics. They are also often applied to agricultural crops as plant growth promoters and biofungicides. In recent years however, some *Trichoderma* spp have emerged as important opportunistic pathogens in patients with compromised immunity and those on peritoneal dialysis [2, 3, 116]. Cases of fatal disseminated disease due to *Trichoderma longibrachiatum* have been reported in patients with hematologic malignancies and in recipients of BMTs and SOTs [116].

Zygomycosis (Mucormycosis)

Zygomycosis and mucormycosis are terms often used interchangeably in the medical literature to describe a group of frequently lethal mold infections that have a predilection for diabetic patients and steroid-treated or severely immunocompromised individuals [117-119]. The majority of human infections are due to fungi mostly belonging to the genera (principal species) *Rhizopus* (*R. arrhizus*), *Mucor* (*M. circinelloides*), *Rhizomucor* (*R. pusillus*), *Cunninghamella* (*C. bertholletiae*), and *Absidia* (*A. corymbifera*). Zygomycete infections are less frequent than invasive mycoses caused by *Aspergillus* spp. Incidence figures are difficult to collect as few national studies have been undertaken. However, the annual incidence of zygomycosis in the state of California has been estimated at 1.7 infections/million individuals based on a sample study performed in three counties [2, 3, 117-119]. Unfortunately, when they do occur, infections due to these agents are generally acute and rapidly progressive with mortality rates of 70-100% [120]. The molds that cause entomophthoramycosis also belong to the class Zygomycetes and comprise *Conidiobolus* spp. and *Basidiobolus* spp. They principally cause nasal, facial and other subcutaneous infections, which may be persistent but rarely disseminate. These are rarely encountered outside of West Africa, India and Central and South America [2, 3, 118, 119].

The infectious spores are initially inhaled before they establish an infection in the sinuses. Other less common routes of acquisition include the intestinal tract following ingestion or by inoculation through breached skin. As zygomycosis is less common than IA, it is believed that Zygomycetes is less virulent [118, 119]. In a study which has reviewed 929 cases of zygomycosis that has been reported up until 2004, the two major risk factors were type 2 diabetes mellitus and malignancy [121]. Whereas rhinocerebral zygomycosis was more commonly associated with diabetes, pulmonary infections occurred more frequently in patients with malignancy. Multivariate analysis has revealed that independent risk factors for increased mortality included disseminated infection. Antifungal therapy and surgery were independently associated with decreased risks of mortality [122]. In a retrospective review of 15 patients with zygomycosis diagnosed at a non-oncology tertiary referral centre between 1999 and 2004 [123], several pertinent observations were made. In that, 9/16 episodes were associated with diabetes mellitus, whereas trauma, vascular disease, steroid therapy and neutropenia were lesser contributory conditions. Ten episodes were due to *Rhizopus* spp. and six were due to *Mucor* spp. Most common infection occurred as wound-related, rhinocerebral, pulmonary, and peritoneal infections; mortality rates were about 25%. Surgical intervention was associated with a trend towards reduced mortality but the numbers were too small to allow statistical significance to be reached. Three patients who further received hyperbaric oxygen therapy were among those who survived. Seven of 12 survivors were left with severe physical or other forms of disability [123]. A significant increase in the incidence of zygomycosis between 2000 and 2003 was attributed to increased use of voriconazole [124,125].

Dematiaceous Molds (Phaeohyphomycosis)

Phaeohyphomycosis describes infections caused by pigmented thick-walled dematiaceous fungi, which comprises a long list of taxonomically diverse group of organisms. The organisms are generally characterized by the presence of a pale brown to dark melanin-like pigment in the cell wall. They may cause a variety of cutaneous and subcutaneous infections in immunocompetent hosts and invasive or disseminated infections in both immunocompetent and immunocompromised hosts [2, 3, 5, 126, 127]. The number of dematiaceous molds reported to be etiologic agents of phaeohyphomycosis continues to grow and several of them appear to be neurotropic [5, 56, 127]. This group includes *Cladophialophora bantiana*, *Bipolaris spicifera*, *Exophiala* spp., *Wangiella dermatitidis*, *Ramichloridium obovoideum*, and *Chaetomium atrobrunneum* [127]. Brain abscess is the most common CNS presentation. While *Bipolaris* spp. and *Exerohilum rostratum* infections initially present as sinusitis, they could extend into the CNS [2, 56, 127, 128].

Histoplasmosis

Histoplasmosis, also known as Darling's disease, is a mycotic disease caused by the dimorphic fungus *Histoplasma capsulatum*. Histoplasmosis is primarily a pulmonary disease with the soil as its environmental reservoir. There are two varieties of *H. capsulatum* that are pathogenic to humans, *H. capsulatum* var. *capsulatum* and *H. capsulatum* var. *duboisii*; a third variety, *H. capsulatum* var. *farciminosum*, is an equine pathogen, [129, 130]. *H. capsulatum* var. *capsulatum* occurs most commonly in North and Central America and in Europe; the organism exists in other area around the world as well (129, 130]. *H. capsulatum* var. *duboisii* exists in Africa and cases reported in Africa and Europe refer to patients of African descent. In the US, *H. capsulatum* is endemic in the Mississippi and Ohio River valleys and some localized mid-eastern foci. Soil containing large amounts of bird or bat guano supports the growth of the mold [130]. Humans acquire *H. capsulatum* infections during day-to-day activities in areas where *H. capsulatum* is highly endemic or in the course of occupational and or recreational activities that disrupt the soil or accumulated dirt in old buildings, on bridges, or in caves where bats have roosted [129,130]. Most individuals with histoplasmosis are asymptomatic; if symptoms are to appear however, they start within 3-17 days (average is 13 days) post exposure. Most affected individuals have clinically silent manifestations and show no apparent ill effects [129,130]. The acute phase of histoplasmosis is characterized by non-specific respiratory symptoms, often cough or flu-like symptoms. Chest X-ray findings are normal in 40–70% of cases. Disseminated histoplasmosis affects multiple organ systems and is fatal unless treated. Severe infections can cause hepatosplenomegaly, lymphoadenopathy, and adrenal gland enlargement. Ocular histoplasmosis damages the retina of the eye and scar tissue left on the retina can cause leakage and loss of vision. Immunosuppressed patients who fail to mount effective CMI against the organism are likely to manifest symptomatic disease during the period of acute dissemination (table 1.5) [129,130].

Table 1.5. Common risk factors for disseminated histoplasmosis

Age (infants)
AIDS
Hematologic malignancies
Solid organ transplants
Hematopoietic stem cell transplant
Immunosuppressive agents
Corticosteroids
Tumor necrosis factor antagonists
Congenital T-cell deficiencies
Gamma interferon receptor deficiency
Hyper-immunoglobulin M syndrome

Less common, yet apparently reemerging fungal diseases such as coccidioidomycosis [131], paracoccidioidomycosis [132], blastomycosis and other unusual fungal and pseudofungal infections [133], though not touched upon in this review, will no doubt draw more attention in the near future.

REFERENCES

[1] Upton A, Marr AK. (2006). Emergence of opportunistic mold infections in the hematopoietic stem cell transplant patient. *Curr. Infect. Dis. Rep.*, 8, 434-441.

[2] Richardson M, Lass-Florl C. (2008). Changing epidemiology of systemic fungal infections. *Clin. Microbiol. Infect.*, 14 (Suppl. 4), 5-24.

[3] Pfaller MA, Diekema DJ. (2004). Rare and emerging opportunistic fungal pathogens: concern for resistance beyond *Candida albicans* and *Aspergillus fumigatus*. *J. Clin. Microbiol.*, 42, 4419-4431.

[4] Cuenca-Estrella M, Bernal-Martinez L, Buitrago MJ, Castelli MV, Gomez-Lopez A, Zaragoza O, Rodriguez-Tudela JL. (2008). Update on the epidemiology and diagnosis of invasive fungal infection. *Inter. J .Antimicrobial Agents*, 32 (Suppl. 2), 143-147.

[5] Caston-Osorio JJ, Rivero A, Torre-Cisneros J. (2008). Epidemiology of invasive fungal infection. *Inter. J. Antimicrobial. Agents*, 32 (Suppl. 2), 103-109.

[6] Pfaller MA, Diekema DJ. (2007). Epidemiology of invasive candidiasis: a persistent public health problem. *Clin. Microbiol. Rev.*, 20, 133-163.

[7] Soni N, Wagstaff A. (2005). Fungal infection. *Curr Anaesthesia Crit Care*, 16, 231-241.

[8] Liu X, Liu H, Guo Z, Luan W. (2006). Association of asymptomatic oral candidal carriage, oral candidiasis and CD4+ lymphocyte count in HIV-positive patients in China. *Oral. Dis.*, 12, 41-44.

[9] Abu-Elteen KH, Hamad MA, Salah, SA. (2006). Prevalence of oral *Candida* infections in diabetic patients. *Bahrain Med. Bull*, 28, 12-17.

[10] Ferrer J. (2000). Vaginal candidiasis: epidemiology and etiological factors. *Intl. J. Gynecol. Obstet.*, 71, 521-527.

[11] Enoch DA, Ludlam HA, Brown NM. (2006). Invasive fungal infections: a review of epidemiology and management options. *J. Med. Microbiol.*, 55, 809-818.

[12] Pirotta MV, Garland M. (2006). Genital *Candida* species detected in samples from women in Melbourne, Australia, before and after treatment with antibiotics *J. Clin. Microbiol.*, 44, 3213-4217.

[13] Beigi RH, Meyn LA, Moore DM, Krohn MA, Hillier SL. (2004). Vaginal yeast colonization in non-pregnant women: A Longitudinal Study. *Obstet. Gynecol.*, 104, 926-930.

[14] Hamad M, Muta'eb E, Abu-Shaqra Q, Fraij A, Abu-Elteen K, Yasin SR. (2006). Utility of the oestrogen-dependent vaginal candidiasis murine

model in evaluating the efficacy of various therapies against vaginal *Candida albicans* infection. *Mycoses*, 49, 104-108.

[15] deLeon EM, Jacober SJ, Sobel JD, Foxman, B. (2002). Prevalence and risk factors for vaginal *Candida* colonization in women with type 1 and type 2 diabetes. *BMC Infect Dis.*, 2, 1.

[16] MacCallum D. (2007). *Candida albicans*: New insights in infection, disease, and treatment, In: Kevin Kavanaugh, editor. New Insights in Medical Mycology, Springer, The Netherlands, 99- 129.

[17] Davies AN, Brailsford SR, Beighton D. (2006). Oral candidiasis in patients with advanced cancer. *Oral. Oncol.*, 42, 698-702.

[18] Abu-Elteen KH, Abu-Elteen RM.(1998).The prevalence of *Candida albicans* populations in the mouths of complete denture wearers. *New Microbiol.*, 21, 41-48.

[19] Sánchez-Vargas LO, Ortiz-López NG, Villar M, Moragues MD, Aguirre JM, Cashat-Cruz M, Lopez-Ribot JL, Gaitán-Cepeda LA, Quindós G. (2005). Oral *Candida* Isolates Colonizing or Infecting Human Immunodeficiency Virus-Infected and Healthy Persons in Mexico, *J. Clin. Microbiol.*, 43, 4159-4162.

[20] Hamad M, Abu-Elteen KH, Ghaleb M. (2004). Estrogen-dependent induction of vaginal candidiasis in naïve mice. *Mycoses*, 47, 304-309.

[21] Abu-Elteen KH. (2001). Increased incidence of vulvovaginal candidiasis caused by Candida glabrata in Jordan. *Jpn J. Infect. Dis.*, 54, 103-107.

[22] Ray D, Goswami R, Banerjee U, Dadhwal V, Goswami D, Mandal P, Sreenivas V, Kochupillai N. (2007). Prevalence of *Candida glabrata* and its response to boric acid vaginal suppositories in comparison with oral fluconazole in patients with diabetes and vulvovaginal candidiasis. *Diabetes Care*, 30, 312-317.

[23] Wisplinghoff H, Bischoff T, Tallent SM, Seifert H, Wenzel RP, Edmond MB. (2004). Nosocomial bloodstream infections in US hospitals: Analysis of 24,179 cases from a prospective nationwide surveillance study. *Clin. Infect. Dis.*, 39, 309-317.

[24] Clark TA, Hajjeh RA. (2004). Recent trends in the epidemiology of invasive mycoses. *Curr. Opin. Infect. Dis.*, 17, 511-515.

[25] Pfaller MA, Pappas PG, Wingard JR. (2006).Invasive fungal pathogens: current epidemiological trends. *Clin. Infect. Dis.*, 43 (Suppl. 1), S3-14.

[26] Tortorano AM, Kibbler C, Peman J, Bernhardt H, Klingspor L, Grillot R. (2006). Candidemia in Europe: epidemiology and resistance. *Int. J. Antimicrob. Agents*, 27, 359-366.

[27] Bougnuox ME, Kac G, Aegerter P, Fagan JY. (2008). Candidemia and candiduria in criticially ill patients admitted to intensive care units in France: incidence, molecular diversity, management and outcome. *Intensive Care Med.*, 34, 292-299.

[28] Vardaka KZ, Michalopoulos A, Kiriakidou KG, Siampl EP, Samonis G, Falagas ME. (2009). Candidemia: incidence, risk factors, characteristics and outcomes in immunocompetent critically ill patients. *Clin. Microbiol. Infect.*, 15, 289-292.

[29] Chow JK, Golan Y, Ruthazerm R, Karchmer A, Garmeli Y, Lichtenberg D, Chawla V, Young JA, Hadley S. (2008). Risk factors for albicans and non albicans candidemia in the intensive care unit. *Crit. Care Med.*, 36, 1993-1998.

[30] Hajjeh RA, Sofair AN, Harrison LH, Lyon GM, Arthington-Skaggs BA, Mirza SA, Phelan M, Morgan J, Lee-Yang W, Ciblak MA, Benjamin LE, Thompson Sanza L, Huie S, Yeo SF, Brandt ME, Warnock DW. (2004). Incidence of bloodstream infections due to *Candida* species and in vitro susceptibilities of isolates collected from 1998 to 2000 in a population-based active surveillance program. *J. Clin. Microbiol.*, 42, 1519-1527.

[31] Pfaller MA, Diekema DJ. (2004). Twelve years of fluconazole in clinical practice: global trends in species distribution and fluconazole susceptibility of bloodstreamisolates of *Candida*. *Clin. Microbiol. Infect.*, 10 (Suppl.1), 11-23.

[32] Bassetti M, Filippo A, Laura N, Emanuele M, Maria Pia M, Michele M, Barbara R, Franco BP, Giancarlo I, Claudio V. (2009). Incidence of candidemia and relationship with fluconazole use in an intensive care unit. *J. Antimicrob. Chemother*, 64(3), 625-629.

[33] Fridkin SK, Kaufman D, Edwards JR, Shetty S, Horan T. (2006). Changing incidence of *Candida* bloodstream infections among NICU patients in the United States: 1995–2004. *Pediatrics*, 117, 1680-1687.

[34] Pasqualotto AC, Rosa DD, Medeiros LR, Severo LC. (2006). Candidemia and cancer: patients are not all the same. *BMC Infect. Dis.*, 6, 50-56.

[35] Peman J, Bosch M, Canton E, Viudes A, Jarque I, Gomez-Garcia M, Garcia-Martinez JM, Gobernado M. (2008). Fungemia due to *Candida guilliermondii* in a pediatric and adult population during a 12-year period. *Diag Microbiol. Infect. Dis.*, 60: 109-112.

[36] Almirante B, Rodríguez D, Park, BJ, Cuenca-Estrella M, Planes AM, Almela M, Mensa J, Sanchez F, Ayats J, Gimenez M, Saballs P, Fridkin

SK, Morgan J, Rodriguez-Tudela JL, Warnock DW, Pahissa A, the Barcelona Candidemia Project Study Group. (2005). Epidemiology and predictors of mortality in cases of *Candida* bloodstream infection: results from population-based surveillance, Barcelona, Spain, from 2002 to 2003. *J. Clin. Microbiol.*, 43, 1829-1835.

[37] Arendrup MC, Fuursted K, Gahrn-Hansen B, Jensen IM, Knudsen JD, Lundgren B, Schønheyder HC, Tvede M. (2005). Semi-national surveillance of fungemia in Denmark: notably high rates of fungemia and numbers of isolates with reduced azole susceptibility. *J. Clin. Microbiol.*, 43, 4434-4440.

[38] Malani A, Hmoud J, Chiu,L, Carver PL, Bielaczyc A, Kauffman CA. (2005). *Candida glabrata* fungemia: experience in a tertiary care center. *Clin. Infect. Dis.*, 41, 975-981.

[39] Shao PL, Huang LM, Hsueh PR. (2007). Recent advances and challenges in the treatment of invasive fungal infections. Inter. *Antimicrob Agents*, 30, 487-495.

[40] Hope W, Morton A, Eisen DP. (2002). Increase in prevalence of nosocomial non-*Candida albicans* candidemia and the association of *Candida krusei* with fluconazole use. *J. Hosp. Infect.* 50, 56-65.

[41] Hammarskjold F, Wallen G, Malmvall BE. (2006). Central venous catheter infections at a county hospital in Sweden: a prospective analysis of colonization, incidence of infection and risk factors. *Acta Anaesthesiol Scand*, 50, 451-460.

[42] Kojic EM, Darouiche RO. (2004). *Candida* infections of medical devices. *Clin. Microbiol. Rev.*, 17, 255-267.

[43] Bicanic T, Harrison TS. (2004). Cryptococcal meningitis. *British Med. Bull*, 72, 99-118.

[44] Subramanian S, Mathai D. (2005). Clinical manifestations and management of cryptococcal infection. *J. Postgrad. Med.*, 51(Suppl 1), 21-26.

[45] Mitchell TG, Perfect JR. (1995). Cryptococcosis in the era of AIDS-100 years after the discovery of *Cryptococcus neoformans*. *Clin. Microbiol. Rev.*, 8, 515-548.

[46] Fraser JA, Giles SS, Wenink EC, Geunes-Boyer SG, Wright JR, Diezmann S, Allen A, Stajichm JE, Dietrich FS, Perfect JR, Heitman J (2005). Same-sex mating and the origin of the Vancouver Island *Cryptococcus gattii* outbreak. *Nature*, 437, 1360-1364.

[47] Morrow CA, Fraser JA. (2009). Sexual reproduction and dimorphism in the pathogenic basidiomycetes, *FEMS Yeast Res.*, 9(2), 161-77.

[48] Casadevall A, Steenbergen JN, Nosanchuk JD. (2003). 'Ready-made' virulence and ' dual use' virulence factors in pathogenic environmental fungi- the *Cryptococcus neoformans* paradigm. *Curr. Opin. Microbiol.*, 6, 332-337.

[49] Levitz SM, Nong S, Seetoo K, Harrison TS, Speizer R, Simons E. (1999). *Cryptococcus neoformans* resides in an acidic phagolysosome of human macrophages. *Infect. Immun.*, 67, 885-890.

[50] Khawcharoenporn T, Apisarnthanarak A, Mundy LM. (2007). Treatment of cryptococcosis in the setting of HIV co-infection. *Expert Rev. Anti Infect. Ther.*, 5, 1019-1030.

[51] Mirza SA, Phelan M, Rimland D. (2003). The changing epidemiology of cryptococcosis: an update from population-based active surveillance in 2 large metropolitan areas,1992-2000. *Clin. Infect. Dis.*, 36, 789-794.

[52] Qazzafi Z, Thiruchunapalli D, Birkenhead D, Bell D. Sandoe JA. (2007). Invasive Cryptococcus neoformans infection in an asplenic patient. *J. Infect.*, 55, 566-568.

[53] Pappas PG, Perfect JR, Cloud GA, Larsen RA, Pankey GA, Lancaster DJ, Henderson H, Kauffman CA, Haas DW, Saccente M, Hamill RJ, Holloway MS, Warren RM, Dismukes WE. (2001). Cryptococcosis in human immunodeficiency virus- negative patients in the era of effective azole therapy. *Clin. Infect. Dis.*, 33, 690-699.

[54] Khawcharoenporn T, Apisarnthanarak A, Mundy LM. (2007). Non-neoformans cryptococcal infections: a systematic review. *Infection*, 35, 51-58.

[55] Lindberg J, Hagen F, Laurson A, Stenderup J, Boekhout T. (2007). *Cryptococcus gattii* risk for tourists visiting Vancouver Island, Canada. *Emerg. Infect. Dis.*, 13, 178-179.

[56] Walsh TJ, Groll A, Hiemenz J, Flemming R, Roilides E, Anaissie E. (2004). Infections due to emerging and uncommon medically important fungal pathogens. *Clin. Microbiol. Infect.*, 10 (Suppl. 1), 48-66

[57] Kontoyiannis DP, Torres HA, Chagua M. (2004). Trichosporonosis in a tertiary care cancer center: risk factors, changing spectrum and determinants of outcome. *Scand J. Infect. Dis.*, 36, 564-569.

[58] Girmenia C, Pagano L, Martino B, D'Antonio D, Fanci R, Specchia G, Melillo L, Buelli M, Pizzarelli G, Venditti M, Martino P, the GIMEMA Infection Program (2005). Invasive infections caused by *Trichosporon* species and *Geotrichum capitatum* in patients with hematological malignancies: a retrospective multicenter study from Italy and review of literature. *J. Clin. Microbiol.*, 43, 1818-1828.

[59] Makela P, Leaman D, Sobel JD. (2003). Vulvovaginal trichosporonosis. *Infect Dis Obtet Gynecol*, 11, 131-133.

[60] Flemming R V, Walsh TJ, Anaissie EJ. (2002). Emerging and less common fungal pathogens. *Infect. Dis. Clin. N. Am.*, 16, 915-933.

[61] Middelhoven WG. (2003). Identification of clinically relevant *Trichosporon* species. *Mycoses*, 46, 7-11.

[62] Marty FM, Barouch DH, Coakley EP, Baden LR. (2003). Disseminated trichosporonosis caused by *Trichosporon loubieri*. *J. Clin. Microbiol.*, 41, 5317-5320.

[63] Hahner D, Kirschner R, Piepenbring M, Schofer H. (2008). First isolation of the anamorphic basidiomycetous yeast *Trichosporon faecale* in Germany, from the skin of a patient with tinea pedis. *Mycopathologia*, 165, 149-153.

[64] Padhye A, Verghese S, Ravichandran P, Balamurugan G, Hall L, Padmaja P, Fernandez MC. (2003). *Trichosporon loubieri* infection in a patient with adult polycystic kidney disease. *J. Clin. Microbiol.*, 41, 479-482.

[65] Hickey PW, Sutton DA, Fothergill AW, Rinaldi MG, Wickes BL, Schmidt HJ, Walsh TJ. (2009). *Trichosporon mycotoxinivorans*: Anovel respiratory pathogen in patients with cystic fibrosis. *J. Clin. Microbiol.*, 47 (10), 3091-3097

[66] Nishiura Y, Nakagawa-Yoshida K, Suga M, Shinoda T, Gueho E, Ando M. (1997). Assignment and serotyping of *Trichosporon* species: the causative agents of summer-type hypersensitivity pneumonitis. *J. Med. Vet. Mycol.*, 35, 45-52.

[67] Sugita T, Nishikawa A, Ikeda R, Sakashita H, Sakai Y, Yoshizawa Y. (1998). First report of *Trichosporon ovoides* isolated from the home summer-type hypersensitivity pneumonitis patient. *Microbiol. Immunol.*, 42, 475-478.

[68] Lo Re V, Fishman NO, Nachamkin I. (2003). Recurrent catheter- related *Rhodotorula rubra* infection. *Clin. Microbiol. Infect.*, 9, 897-900.

[69] Zaas A.K, Boyce M, Schell W, Alexander lodge B, Miller JL, Perfect JR. (2003). Risk of fungemia due to *Rhodotorula* and antifungal susceptibility testing of *Rhodotorula* isolates. *J. Clin. Microbiol.*, 41, 5233-5235.

[70] Thakur K, Singh G, Agarwal S, Rani L. (2007). Meningitis caused by *Rhodotorula rubra* in an human immunodeficiency virus infected patient. *Indian J. Med. Microbiol.*, 25, 166-168.

[71] Hsueh PR, Teng LJ, Ho SW, Luh KT. (2003). Catheter- related sepsis due to *Rhodotorula glutinis*. *J. Clin. Microbiol.*, 41, 857-859.

[72] Shinde RS, Mantur BG, Patil G, Parande MV, Parande AM. (2008). Meningitis due to *Rhodotorula glutinis* in an HIV infected patients. *Indian J. Med. Microbiol.*, 26, 375-377.

[73] Baradkar VP, Kumar S. (2008). Meningitis caused by *Rhodotorula mucilaginosa* in human immunodeficiency virus seropositive patient. *Ann. Indian Acad. Neurol.*, 11, 245-247.

[74] Riedel DJ, Johnson JK, Forrest GN. (2007). *Rhodotorula glutinis* fungemia in a liver-kidney transplant patient. *Transplant Infect. Dis.*, 10, 197-200.

[75] Fung HB, Martyn CA, Shahidi A, Brown ST. (2008). *Rhodotorula mucilaginosa* lymphadenitis in an HIV- infected patient. *Inter. J. Infect. Dis.*, 13, e27-e29.

[76] De Almeida G, Costa SF, Melhem M, Motta AL, Szeszs MW, Miyashita F, Pierrotti LC, Rossi F, Burattini MN.(2008). *Rhodotorula* spp. isolated from blood cultures: clinical and microbiological aspects. *Med. Mycol.*, 46, 547-556.

[77] Tuon FF, de Almeida GM, Costa SF. (2007). Central venous catheter-associated fungemia due to *Rhodotorula* spp—a systematic review. *Med. Mycol.*, 45: 441–447.

[78] Bouza E, MunozP. (2004). Invasive infection caused by *Blastoschizomyces capitatus* and *Scedosporium* spp. *Clin. Microbiol. Infect.*, 10(Suppl. 1), 76-85.

[79] Martino R, Salavert M, Parody R, Tomas JF, de la Camara R, Vazquez L, Jarque I, Prieto E, Sastre JL, Gadea I, Peman J, Sierra J. (2004). *Blastoschizomyces capitatus* infection in patients with leukemia: report of 26 cases. *Clin. Infect. Dis.*, 38, 335-341.

[80] Maschmeyer G, Haas A, Cornely OA. (2007). Invasive aspergillosis: epidemiology, diagnosis and management in immunocompromised patients. *Drugs*, 67, 1567-1601.

[81] Singh N, Paterson DL. (2005). *Aspergillus* infections in transplant recipients. *Clin. Microbiol. Rev.*, 18, 44-69.

[82] Denning DW. (1998). Invasive aspergillosis. *Clin. Infect. Dis.*, 26, 781-805.

[83] Rosenhagen M, Feldhues R, Schmidt J, Hoppe-Tichy T, Geiss HK. (2009). A risk profile for invasive aspergillosis in liver transplant recipients. *Infection*, 37, 313-319.

[84] Denning D.W. (1995). Issues in the management of invasive aspergillosis. *Ann. Med. Interne*, 146, 106-110.

[85] Verweij PE, Denning DW. (1997). Diagnostic and therapeutic strategies for invasive aspergillosis. *Respir. Crit. Care Med.*, 18:203-215.

[86] Patterson TF. (2005). Advances and challenges in management of invasive mycoses. *Lancet*, 366, 1013-1025.

[87] Nivoix Y, Velten M, Letscher-Bru V, Moghaddam A, Natarajan- Ame S, Fohrer C, Lioure B, Bilger K, Lutun P, Marcellin L, Launoy A, Freys G, Bergerat JP, Herbrecht R. (2008). Factors associated with overall and attributable mortality in invasive aspergillosis. *Clin. Infect. Dis.*, 47, 1176-1184.

[88] Marr KA, Carter RA, Crippa F, Wald A, Corey L. (2002). Epidemiology and outcome of mold infections in hematopoietic stem cell transplant recipients. *Clin. Infect. Dis.*, 34, 909-917.

[89] Pagano L, Caira M, Nosari A, Van Lint MT, Candoni A, Offidani M, Aloisi T, Irrera G, Bonini A, Picardi M, Caramatti C, Invernizzi R, Mattei D, Melillo L, de Waure C, Reddiconto G, Fianchi L, Valentini CG, Girmenia C, Leone G, Aversa F. (2007). Fungal Infections in Recipients of Hematopoietic Stem Cell Transplants: Results of the SEIFEM B-2004 Study—Sorveglianza Epidemiologica Infezioni Fungine Nelle Emopatie Maligne. *Clin. Infect. Dis.*, 45, 1161-1170.

[90] Martino R, Subirá M, Rovira M, Solano C, Vázquez L, Sanz GF, Urbano-Ispizua A, Brunet S, De la Cámara R. (2002). Invasive fungal infections after allogeneic peripheral blood stem cell transplantation: incidence and risk factors in 395 patients. *Br. J. Hematol.*, 116, 475-482.

[91] Upton A, Kirby KA, Carpenter P, Boeckh M, Marr KA. (2007). Invasive aspergillosis following hematopoietic cell transplantation: Outcomes and prognostic factors associated with mortality. *Clin. Infect. Dis.*, 44: 531-540.

[92] Gavalda J, Len O, San Juan R, Aguado JM, Fortun J, Lumbreras C, Moreno A, Munoz P, Blanes M, Ramos A, Rufi G, Gurgui M, Torre-Cisneros T, Montejo, M., Cuenca-Estrella M, Rodriguez-Tudela JL, Pahissa A, RESITRA -Spanish Network for Research on Infection in Transplantation- (2005). Risk factors for invasive Aspergillosis in solid-organ transplant recipients: A case-control study. *Clin. Infect. Dis.*, 41, 52-59.

[93] Cornillet A,Camus C, Nimubona S, Gandemer V, Tattevin P, Belleguic C, Chevrier S, Meunier C, Lebert C, Aupée M, Caulet-Maugendre S, Faucheux M, Lelong B, Leray E, Guiguen C, Gangneux JP. (2006).

Comparison of Epidemiological, Clinical, and Biological Features of Invasive Aspergillosis in Neutropenic and Non-neutropenic Patients: A 6-Year Survey. *Clin. Infect. Dis.*, 43, 577-584.

[94] Meersseman W, Lagrou K, Maertens J, Van Wijngaerden E. (2007). Invasive Aspergillosis in the Intensive Care Unit. *Clin. Infect. Dis.*, 45, 205-216.

[95] Howard SJ, Cerar D, Anderson MJ, Albarrag A, Fisher MC, Pasqualotto AC, Laverdiere M, Arendrup MC, Perlin DS, Denning DW. (2009). Frequency and evolution of azole resistance in Aspergillus fumigatus associated with treatment failure. *Emerg. Infect. Dis.*, 15: 1068-1076.

[96] Steinbach WJ, Benjamin DK Jr, Kontoyiannis DP, Perfect JR, Lutsar I, Marr KA, Lionakis MS, Torres HA, Jafri H, Walsh TJ. (2004). Infections Due to *Aspergillus terreus:* A Multicenter Retrospective Analysis of 83 Cases. *Clin. Infect. Dis.*, 39, 192-198.

[97] Lass-Florl C, Griff K, Mayr A, Petzer A, Gastl G, Bonatti H, Freund M, Kropshofer G, Dierich M, Nachbaur D. (2005). Epidemiology and outcome of infections due to Aspergillus terreus: 10-year single centre experience. *Br. J. Hematol.*, 131, 201-207.

[98] Hedayati MT, Pasqualotto AC, Warn PA, Bowyer P, Denning DW. (2007). *Aspergillus flavus*: human pathogen, allergen and mycotoxin producer. *Microbiology*, 153, 1677-1692.

[99] Balajee SA, Gribskov JL, Hanley E, Nickle D, Marr KA. (2006). *Aspergillus lentulus* sp. nov., a new sibling species of *A. fumigatus*. *Eukaryot Cell*, 4, 625-632.

[100] Ando T, Moriya A, Shibuya K. (2008). Aspergillosis. *Nippon Rinsho*, 66, 2345-2349.

[101] Abu-Elteen KH, Hamad M. (2007). Novel antifungal therapies. In: Kevin Kavanagh, editor. New Insights in Medical Mycology, Springer, The Netherlands, 69-98.

[102] Cortez KJ, Roilides E, Quiroz-Telles F, Meletiadis J, Antachopoulos C, Knudsen T, Buchanan W, Milanovich J, Sutton DA, Fothergill A, Rinaldi MG, Shea YR, Zaoutis T, Kottilil S, Walsh TJ. (2008). Infections caused by *Scedosporium* spp. *Clin. Microbiol. Rev.*, 21, 157-197.

[103] Nucci M, Anaissie E. (2007). Fusarium infections in immunocompromised patients. *Clin. Microbiol. Rev.*, 20, 695-704.

[104] Mellinghoff IK, Winston DJ, Mukwaya G, Schiller GJ. (2002). Treatment of *Scedosporium apiospermum* brain abscesses with posaconazole. *Clin. Infect. Dis.*, 34, 1648-1650.

[105] Nesky MA, McDougal C, Peacock JE Jr. (2000). *Pseudallescheria boydii* brain abscess successfully treated with voriconazole and surgical drainage: case report and literature review of central nervous system pseudallescheriosis. *Clin. Infect. Dis.*, 31, 673-677.

[106] Perlroth J, Choi B, Spellberg B. (2007). Nosocomial fungal infections: epidemiology, diagnosis, and treatment. *Med. Mycol.*, 45, 321-346.

[107] Dignani MC, Anaissie E. (2004). Human fusariosis. *Clin. Microbiol. Infect.*, 10 (Suppl 1), 67-75.

[108] Anaissie EJ, Kuchar RT, Rex JH, Francesconi A, Kasai M, Müller FMC, Lozano-Chiu M, Summerbell RC, Dignani MC, Chanock ST, Walsh TJ. (2001). Fusariosis Associated with Pathogenic *Fusarium* Species Colonization of a Hospital Water System: A New Paradigm for the Epidemiology of Opportunistic Mold Infections. *Clin. Infect. Dis.*, 33, 1871-1878.

[109] Nucci M, Anaissie E. (2002). Cutaneous Infection by *Fusarium* Species in Healthy and Immunocompromised Hosts: Implications for Diagnosis and Management. *Infect. Dis.*, 35, 909-920.

[110] Nucci M, Marr KA, Queiroz-Telles F, Martins CA, Trabasso, P, Costa S, Voltarelli JC, Colombo AL, Imhof A, Pasquini R, Maiolino A, Souza CA, Anaissie E. (2004). *Fusarium* Infection in Hematopoietic Stem Cell Transplant Recipients. *Clin. Infect. Dis.*, 38, 1237-1242.

[111] Walsh TJ, Groll A, Hiemenz J, Fleming R, Roilides E, Anaissie E. (2004). Infections due to emerging and uncommon medically important fungal pathogens. *Clin. Microbiol. Infect.*, 10 (Suppl. 1), 48-66.

[112] Schinabeck MK, Ghannoum MA. (2003). Human hyalohyphomycoses: a review of human infections due to *Acremonium* spp., *Paecilomyces* spp., *Penicillium* spp., and *Scopulariopsis* spp. *J. Chemother.,* 15 (suppl 2), 5–15.

[113] Miyakis S, Velegraki A, Delikou S, Parcharidou A, Papadakis V, Kitra V, Papadatos I, Polychronopoulou S.(2006) Invasive Acremonium strictum infection in a bone marrow transplant recipient. *Pediatr. Infect. Dis.*, 25, 273–275.

[114] Pastor FJ, Guarro J. (2006). Clinical manifestations, treatment and outcome of *Paecilomyces lilacinus* infections. *Clin. Microbiol. Infect.*, 12, 948–960.

[115] van Schooneveld T, Freifeld A, Lesiak B, Kalil A, Sutton AD, Iwen *PC. (*2008). *Paecilomyces lilacinus* infection in a liver transplant patient: case report and review of the literature. *Transpl. Infect. Dis.*, 10, 117-122.

[116] Chouaki T, Lavarde V, Lachaud L, Raccurt CP, Hennequin C. (2002). Invasive infections due to *Trichoderma* species: report of 2 cases, findings of in vitro susceptibility testing, and review of the literature. *Clin. Infect. Dis.*, 35, 1360-1367.

[117] Bitar D, Van Cauteren D, Lanternier F, Dannaoui E, Che D, Dromer F, Desenclose GC, Lortholary O. (2009). Increasing incidence of zygomycosis (mucormycosis), France, 1997-2006. *Emerg. Infect. Dis.*, 15: 1395-1401.

[118] Spellberg B, Edwards J Jr, Ibrahim A. (2005). Novel perspectives on mucormycosis: pathophysiology, presentation, and management. *Clin. Microbiol. Rev.*, 18, 556–569.

[119] Chayakulkeeree M, Ghannoum MA, Perfect JR. (2006). Zygomycosis: the re-emerging fungal infection. *Eur J Microbiol Infect Dis*, 25, 215–229.

[120] Gonzalez CE, Rinaldi MG, Sugar AM. (2002). Zygomycosis. *Infect. Dis. Clin. N. Am.*, 16, 895-914.

[121] Roden MM, Zaoutis TE, Buchanan WL, Knudsen TA, Sarkisova TA, Schaufele RL, Sein M, Sein T, Chiou CC, Chu JH, Konotoyiannis AD, Walsh TJ. (2005). Epidemiology and outcome of zygomycosis: a review of 929 reported cases. *Clin. Infect. Dis.*, 41, 634–653.

[122] Rogers T. (2008). Treatment of zygomycosis: current and new options. *J. Antimicrob. Chemother.*, 61(Suppl 1), 35-39.

[123] Sims CR, Ostrosky-Zeichner L. (2007). Contemporary treatment and outcomes of zygomycosis in a non-oncologic tertiary care center. *Arch. Med. Res.*, 38, 90–93.

[124] Trifilio SM, Bennett CL, Yarnold PR, McKoy JM, Parada J, Mehta J, Chamilos G, Palella F, Kennedy L, Mullane K, Tallman MS, Evens A, Scheetz MH, Blum W, Kontoyiannis DP. (2007). Breakthrough zygomycosis after voriconazole administration among patients with hematologic malignancies who receive hematopoietic stem-cell transplants or intensive chemotherapy. *Bone Marrow Transplant*, 39, 425–429.

[125] Almyroudis NG, Sutton DA, Fothergill AW, Rinaldi MG, Kusne S. (2007). *In vitro* susceptibilities of 217 clinical isolates of zygomycetes to conventional and new antifungal agents. *Antimicrob. Agents Chemother.*, 51, 2587–2590.

[126] Negroni R, Helou SH, Petri N, Robles AM, Arechavala A, Bianchi MH. (2004). Case study: posaconazole treatment of disseminated

phaeohyphomycosis due to *Exophiala spinifera*. *Clin. Infect. Dis.*, 38, e15-e20.

[127] Revankar SG, Sutton DA, Rinaldi MG. (2004). Primary central nervous system phaeohyphomycosis: a review of 101 cases. *Clin. Infect. Dis.*, 38, 206-216.

[128] Yehia M, Thomas M, Dilmore H, Van der Merwe W, Dittner I. (2004). Subcutaneous black fungus (phaeohyphomycosis) infection in renal transplant recipients: three cases. *Transplantation*, 77, 140-142.

[129] Kauffman CA. (2007). Histoplasmosis: a clinical and laboratory update. *Clin. Microbiol. Rev.*, 20, 115-132.

[130] Kauffman CA. (2009). Histoplasmosis. *Clin. Chest Med.*, 30, 217-225.

[131] Cox RA, Magee DM. (2004). Coccidioidomycosis: Host response and vaccine development. *Clin. Microbiol. Rev.*, 17, 804-839.

[132] Travassos LR, Goldman G, Taborda C, Puccia R. (2007). Insights in Paracoccidioides barasiliensis pathogenicity. In: Kevin Kavanagh, editor.New Insights in Medical Mycology, Springer, The Netherlands, 241-265.

[133] Pfaller MA, Diekema DJ. (2005). Unusual fungal and pseudofungal infections of humans. *J. Clin. Microbiol.*, 43, 1495-1504.

Chapter 2

TREATMENT OF HUMAN FUNGAL INFECTIONS

Systematic therapy of human fungal infections has started more than a century ago. Potassium iodide was first introduced as an antifungal agent in 1903; this was followed by the introduction of Whitefield's ointment in 1907 and undecylenic acid in the 1940s [reviewed in 1 and references therein]. Garlic extracts (allicin), seed and leaf oils (tea tree, orange, olive and so on), yogurt, benzoic acid, zinc, and selenium were also used during that era. Some of these preparations are still in use as alternative (or more precisely folk) medicines.

Treatment of human fungal infections has certainly come a long way since then. To be sure, in the last 50 years, considerable advances have been made in antifungal chemotherapy through the introduction of a wide array of antifungal drugs to treat most forms of human fungal infections. For example, the poleyne class of antifungal drugs (nystatin and amphotericin B) was first discovered and put to clinical use in the early 1950s. On the heels of that breakthrough, the number of antifungal agents in terms of chemical composition, mechanism of action, and target pathogens has expanded to a considerable degree.

In addition to conventional chemotherapy, several unconventional therapies such as biological inhibitors, oligonucleotides, and probiotics exhibit significant antifungal activity.

Although some of these therapies (probiotics and natural products) fall into the folk medicines category, others fall into the growing list of "potential" or "seriously promising" antifungal therapies.

Conventional Treatment: Chemotherapy

In general terms, antifungal chemotherapy relies on the capacity of various drugs to inhibit or disrupt the synthesis or integrity of cell wall components, plasma membranes, cellular metabolism, fungal proteins, mitotic activity (table 1) [2-4 and references therein] and signaling cascades [5-8].

Table 2.1. Commonly used antifungal drugs

Class	General mechanism of action	Susceptible fungi
Active against cell wall components		
Echinocandins: (caspofungin, micafungin anidulafungin)	inhibit cell wall glucan synthesis by blocking (1,3)-β-D glucan synthase activity	*Candida* species
Nikkomycin and *Aureobasidin*	inhibit chitin synthesis and assembly	*Candida* and *Cryptococcus* species
Active against plasma membrane integrity or synthesis		
Polyenes (amphotericin B and nystatin)	Auto-oxidation of ergosterol and formation of free radicals which compromise plasma membrane integrity and increase permeability	Different species of *Candida, Aspergillus, Histoplasma, Coccidioides, Cryptococcus*, and *Saccharomyces*
Azoles (voriconazole, posaconazole, itraconazole, ravuconazole, and others)	Inhibit ergosterol synthesis by blocking the activity of the P450-dependent enzyme 14 α-demethylase	Different species of *Candida, Aspergillus*, and *Cryptococcus*
Allylamines (terbinafine and naftifine), *Thiocarbamates* (tolnaftate)	Inhibit the activity of squalene epoxidase which is responsible for the cyclization of squalene to lanosterol	Different species of *Aspergillus, Fusarium, Penicillium, Trichoderma, Acremonoim*, and *Arthrographis*
Active against protein synthesis		
Sordarins (sordaricin methyl ester)	Disrupt displacement of tRNA from A site to P site and movement of ribosomes along the mRNA thread by blocking the activity of elongation factor EF2 and the large ribosomal subunit stalk rpPO.	*C. albicans* and *S. cerevisiae*
5-fluorocytosine	Inhibits pyrimidine metabolism by disrupting RNA and protein synthesis	Different species of *Candida, Aspergillus*, and *Cryptococcus*

Antifungal agents currently available for clinical use belong to four major classes: polyenes, azoles, 5-fluorocytosine, and echinocandins. Additional antifungal compounds like allylamines, nikkomycin, aureobasidin, thiocarbamates, sordarins and others are also often available to treat specific forms of mycosis. These drugs differ in many respects regarding structure, water solubility, mode of action, spectrum of activity, and degree of toxicity. Based on the mechanism of action and the degree of selective toxicity, antifungal agents can kill fungal cells (fungicidal) or reversibly inhibit their growth (fungistatic). In terms of activity, antifungal drugs are either broad-spectrum (used against a wide range of fungal species) or narrow-spectrum (target one or few fungal species). Topical antifungal agents are used to treat local infections while systemic antifungal agents are used to treat systemic and disseminated fungal infections. Antifungal agents can be naturally derived (antibiotic) or chemically synthesized (synthetic) compounds. The long history, efforts, and resources dedicated towards the development of new antifungal agents notwithstanding, the number of antifungal drugs approved for clinical use remains limited. Currently, only a dozen or so antifungal drugs are FDA-approved to treat fungal infections in the United States. Although this can be attributed to several compounding factors, the limited number of molecular targets that can set eukaryotic fungi apart from mammalian cells, the enormous complexity and genetic sophistication of pathogenic fungi, and the ability of antifungals to induce resistance and cause side effects bear most of the blame.

Drugs Targeting the Cell Wall

The cell wall is the interface between cells and their environment; cell walls protect against osmotic pressure and control passage of molecules in and out of cells. Therefore, disruption of cell wall integrity or synthesis is detrimental to cell viability and survival. Antifungal agents active against fungal cell wall components (mannans, chitins, α- and β-glucans) are the candins (echinocandin and aminocandin), nikkomycin and aureobasidins. Echinocandins represent a new class of lipopeptides that have proven to be safe and effective against candidiasis when given intravenously. FDA-approved echinocandins (caspofungin, micafungin and anidulafungin; see figure 2.1 below) as well as some related compounds (aminocandin) are effective fungistatic and fungicidal agents owing to their capacity to inhibit glucan synthesis by blocking the activity of (1,3)-β-D glucan synthase.

Echinocandins are very active against *Candida* species; however, other fungal pathogens including *Aspergillus* and *Cryptococcus* species are also susceptible to echinocandin activity. The leading chitin synthesis inhibitor is the fungicidal agent nikkomycin, which is active against the dimorphic fungi *Coccidioides immitis* and *Blactomyces dermatitidis*.

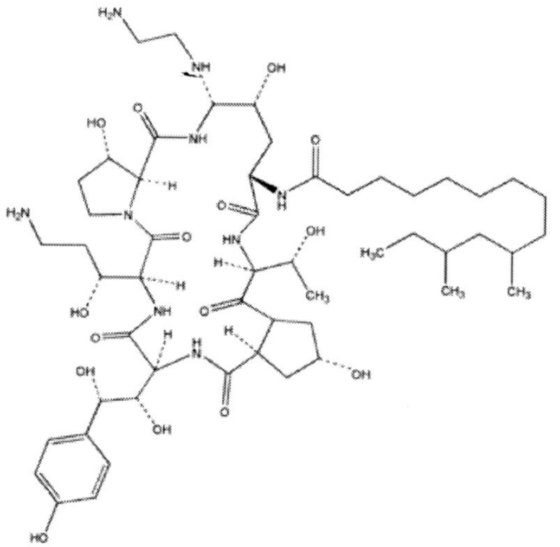

caspofungin

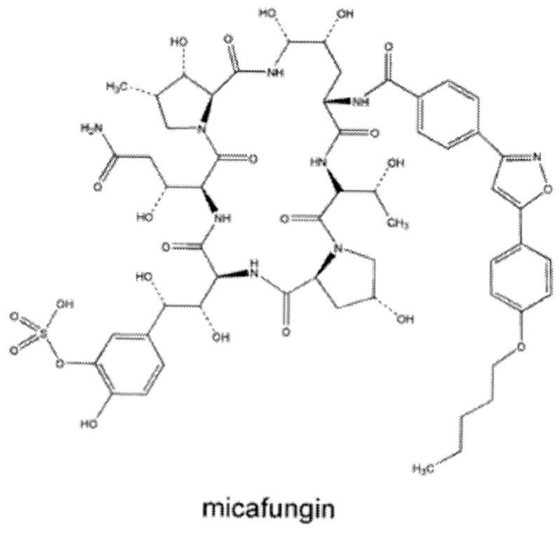

micafungin

Figure 2.1 (Continued)

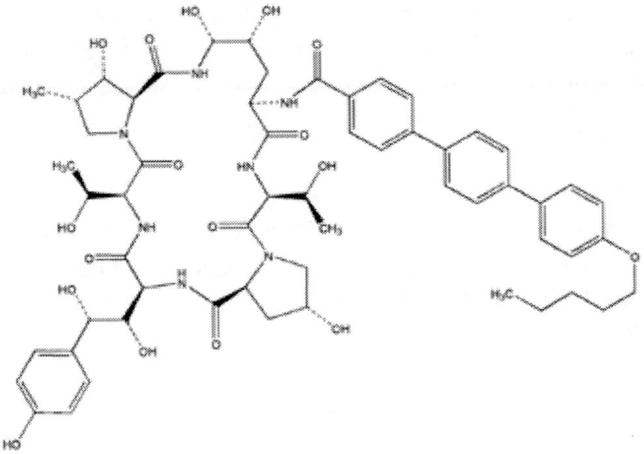

anidulafungin

Figure 2.1. FDA-approved echinocandins.

Aureobasidins alter chitin assembly and sphingolipid synthesis; the drug is mainly active against *Candida* species and *Cryptococcus neoformans* but has some potency against *Histoplasma capsulatum* and *B. dermatitidis*.

Drugs Targeting the Plasma Membrane

Antifungal agents that disrupt plasma membrane synthesis and cellular metabolism remain the most commonly prescribed drugs to treat pre-systemic and systemic fungal infections. These include polyenes, azoles, allylamines and thiocarbamates. Polyenes (amphotericin B or AMB and nystatin or NY) form complexes with and induce auto-oxidation of ergosterol with the subsequent generation of free radicals that disrupt fungal plasma membranes and cause increased permeability and cell death. The development of lipid-based delivery systems (phospholipid vesicles or liposomes and cholesterol esters) of AMB has enhanced the drug's therapeutic index by decreasing toxicity and increasing target specificity. Other lipid formulations like the AMB lipid complex (AMBLC) and the lipid-formulated AMB colloidal dispersion (AMBCD) have also been granted FDA approval for clinical use in the mid 1990s. NY, which binds ergosterol and causes alterations in membrane permeability that lead to cell death, is active against *Candida,*

Aspergillus, Histoplasma species and *Coccidioides immitis*; the drug is relatively safe when administered intravenously. SPA-S-753 a new water soluble polyene active against *Candida*, *Cryptococcus* and *Saccharomyces* species yields higher survival rates, longer survival times and better sterilization of infected organs as compared with the parent molecule (AMB).

Azole and azole derivatives represent a rapidly expanding group of antifungal drugs. Common examples include fluconazole and its derivatives (voriconazole and ravuconazole) itraconazole and its hydroxylated analogue posaconazole (figure 2.2). Voriconazole inhibits ergosterol synthesis by inhibiting P450-dependent 14α-demethylase demethylation in *C. albicans*, *A. fumigatus*, *C. neoformans*, and other dimorphic fungi. Posaconazole is active against different species of *Candida*, *C. neoformans*, *Aspergillus*, *Fusarium*, zygomycetes, and some dematiaceous molds. Ravuconazole is an oral derivative of fluconazole with expanded spectrum of *in vitro* activity. Its inhibitory potency and binding affinity to P-450-dependent 14α-demethylase is similar to that of itraconazole.

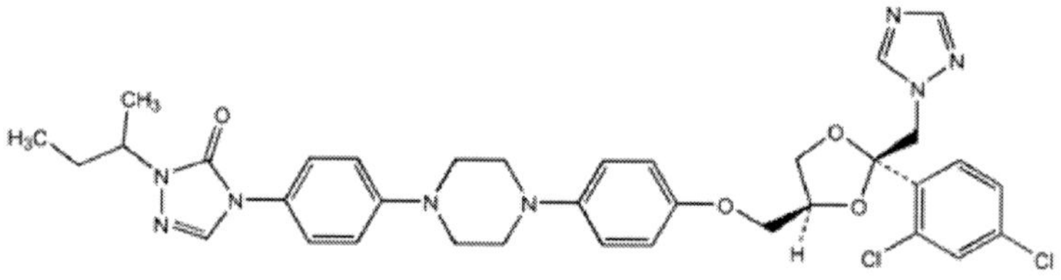

itraconazole

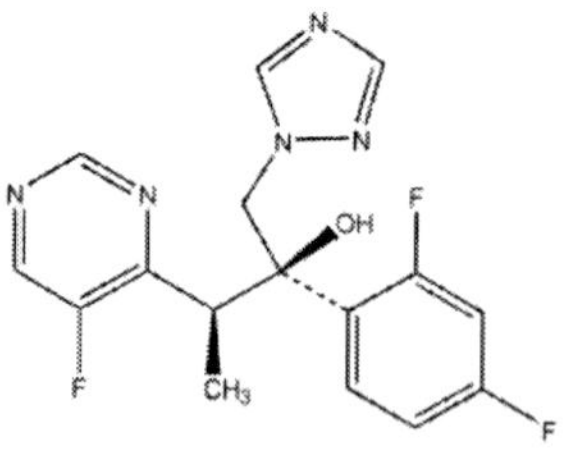

voriconazole

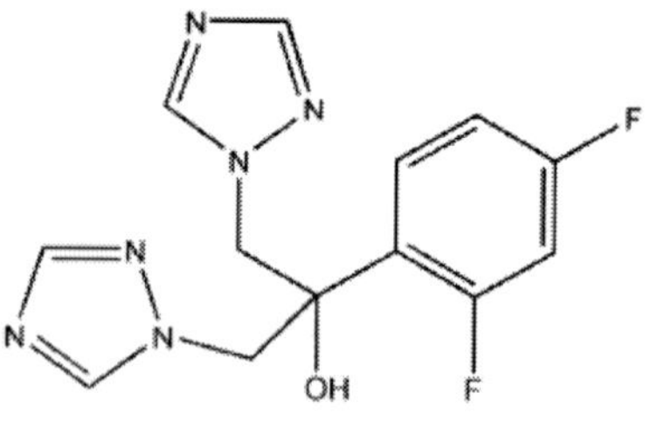

fluconazole

Figure 2.2. Representative examples of azole-based antifungal drugs.

The drug is active against *Candida* species, *A. fumigatus*, *C. neoformans*, hyaline hyphomycetes, dermatophytes, and dematiaceous fungi. The allylamines terbinafine and naftifine and the thiocarbamate tolnaftate are synthetic inhibitors of squalene epoxidase, the enzyme responsible for the cyclization of squalene to lanosterol. They possess fungicidal activity against dermatophytes, *Aspergillus* species, *Fusarium* species, *Penicillium marneffei* and other filamentous fungi. Terbinafine has strong *in vitro* activity against different species of *Penicillium*, *Paecilomyces*, *Trichoderma*, *Acremonoim*, and *Arthrographis*.

Drugs Targeting Protein Synthesis

Antifungal compounds targeting protein synthesis include the sordarins and azosordarins (figure 2.3). Sordarins target elongation factor (EF)2 and the large ribosomal subunit stalk rpPO. Hence they disrupt the displacement of tRNA from A site to P site and block the movement of ribosomes along the mRNA thread.

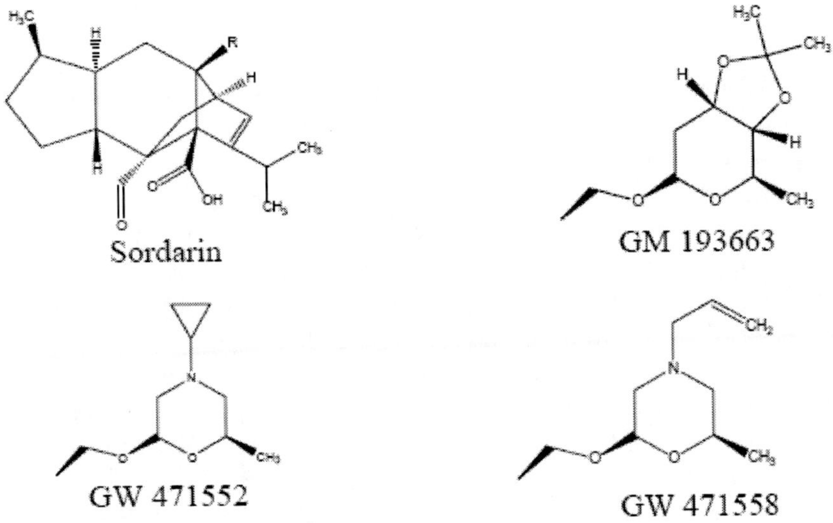

Figure 2.3. Sordarin and some of its derivatives.

Azasordarins target and disrupt polypeptide chain elongation with activity superior to that of sordarins especially in the case of candidiasis. Unlike the classical EF1α and EF2 used by both fungal and mammalian cells for polypeptide chain growth, the discovery of EF3 as a new EF for protein synthesis unique to yeast cells has allowed fungal protein translation to evolve as a desirable target. 5-fluorocytosine (5-FC), which inhibits pyrimidine metabolism by interfering with RNA and protein synthesis, is the sole antimitotic antifungal agent in clinical use. The drug is active against *Candida*, *Aspergillus*, and *Cryptococcus* species as well as dematiaceous fungi that cause chromomycosis (*Phialophora* and *Cladosporium*). Combining 5-FC with various AMB formulations is useful in clearing the cerebrospinal fluid in non-HIV patients infected with cryptococcal meningitis, candidiasis, *Candida* endophthalmitis, renal and hepatosplenic candidiasis, *Candida* thrombophlebitis of the great veins, aspergillosis, and central nervous system (CNS) phaeohyphomycosis.

Cell Signaling Inhibitors

Interruption of cellular signaling cascades is a powerful tool to combat cancers, viral infections, transplant rejection, autoimmunity among other ailments. There is ample evidence to suggest that interruption of signaling cascades is effective against common forms of mycoses (candidiasis, cryptococosis and aspergillosis) [5-9]. Calcineurin inhibitors cyclosporine A (CsA) and Fermentek catalogue number 506 (FK506), the mammalian target of rapamycin (mTOR) inhibitor sirolimus (rapamycin), the heat shock protein 90 (HSP90) inhibitor geldanamycin, the phosphatidylinositol 3-kinase inhibitor wortmannin and the angiogenesis inhibitors fumagillin and ovalicin are all associated with broad spectrum antifungal activity. For instance, the function of calcineurin, a Ca^{2}/calmodulin-dependent phosphatase that plays a role in T cell activation [10-12], can be compromised by the capacity of FK506 or CsA to form drug-protein complexes [13, 14]. In turn, the proliferation and mitotic activity of target cells is halted. As fungi are eukaryotes, calcineurin inhibitors seem to disrupt signaling cascades within fungal cells and halt their growth [5-9]. It must be emphasized that this mode of treatment with regard to fungal infections is still in its infancy; no inhibitor drugs that disrupt signaling cascades in fungal pathogens have been approval for clinical use yet. Though not directly related to this discussion, it is worth noting that work on fungal virulence factors and their inhibitors is becoming a rich source of new therapeutic concepts and candidates to prevent and treat fungal infections. One of the prime examples here is the development of inhibitors to the secreted aspartic proteinase of *C. albicans* [reviewed in 15]. However, like fungal cell signaling inhibitors, this approach is still in the early explorative stage.

No Magic Bullets

Notwithstanding the enormous benefits of antifungal chemotherapy, problems regarding toxic side effects, resistance, variable spectra of activity, inability to fully clear infections, and limited molecular targets persist. To overcome these limitations and make antifungal chemotherapy more appealing to practitioners and patients, ideal antifungals have been sought. Ideal in the sense that they exhibit enhanced potency, broad spectrum of activity, minimized mechanism-based host toxicity, flexible mode of administration, and favorable pharmacokinetics (bioavailability and effective tissue penetration) [6]. In this respect, some of the newer triazoles (posaconazole, ravuconazole, and voriconazole) and echinocandins (anidulafungin, caspofungin, and micafungin) appear to meet some of these requirements. However, reports on the emergence of resistance and the development of toxic side effects in association with the use of these new drugs are beginning to trickle in [16]. Therefore, it seems that developing the ideal "magic bullet" antifungal is more of a hope than a possibility given the inevitable toxicity and resistance consequences of antifungal chemotherapy. On the one hand, the considerable molecular and biochemical resemblance between fungal and host cells, both being eukaryotic, will always be a limiting factor in the process of developing safe, yet selectively toxic, drugs. On the other hand, the sophisticated and flexible genetic makeup of fungi will always be sort of a springboard for fungi to counter the adverse effects of drugs, bounce back, and become resistant to them. In other words, regardless of the chemical composition or delivery system of chemotherapy, improvements on existing antifungals can only go so far to partially address some, but not all, the negative aspects of antifungal chemotherapy.

Unconventional Antifungal Therapies

The diverse means by which different agents tend to kill fungal pathogens or inhibit their growth presents a unique opportunity to develop and test different kinds of molecules as potential antifungal drugs. This coupled with the realization that antifungal chemotherapy will likely continue to be hampered by fungal resistance, toxicity and other problems, preventive and therapeutic alternatives have been sought. Work in this area has shown that numerous oligonucleotides [17, 18], antineoplastics [19-21], biological blockers [22, 23], and probiotics [24, 25] possess significant antifungal activity. Furthermore, long lists of agents and preparations are undergoing rigorous screening and testing as potential antifungals. Although available data regarding specific examples of such agents is promising [17, 18, 22, 23], this approach on the whole is yet to become a significant source of clinically valuable antifungal drugs. Owing to their diverse origins, structures, and mechanisms of action, it is difficult to classify alternative antifungals into any coherent set of categories. For example, while the majority of such agents directly target fungal pathogens, some have immunomodulatory potential. They may come as already in-use drugs, nucleotide sequences, preparations that contain whole or processed micro-organisms and so on.

Drugs and Biological Inhibitors

Deferasirox, an FDA-approved oral iron chelator, is used to reduce chronic iron overload in patients on long-term blood transfusion therapy for anemia. Administration of deferasirox into diabetic ketoacidotic or neutropenic mice with mucormycosis results in improved survival and decreased tissue fungal burden at levels comparable to that of LAMB [26]. Treatment with deferasirox in combination with LAMB significantly enhanced treatment outcome as compared with treatment with either agent alone [26]. Intraperitoneal administration of daucosterol (a beta-sitosterol glycoside) before intravenous challenge with viable *C. albicans* cells induced Th2 protective immunity, prolonged survival and partially cleared kidney fungal load in mice with disseminated candidiasis [27]. Pentraxin 3 (PTX3), a member of the long pentraxins subgroup of the pentraxin family, is an essential component of innate immunity against pulmonary aspergillosis [28]. PTX3 was reported to modulate cytokine production and enhance complement responses to pulmonary aspergillosis. When administered intranasally or parenterally before, during, or after intranasal inoculation with *A. fumigatus* conidia, PTX3 renders mice transplanted with allogeneic bone marrow resistant to aspergillosis at levels equal or superior to that induced by AMB or LAMB [28]. Co-administration of PTX3 with suboptimal doses of either antifungal potentiates therapeutic efficacy associated with accelerated recovery of lung phagocytes and Th cells. Indinavir (IDV), conventionally used as an antiretroviral protease inhibitor (PI), was shown to induce the expansion of splenic CD8α^+ DCs in hosts infected with *C. neoformans* [26]. Upregulated expression of costimulatory molecules (CD40 and CD80) and proinflammatory cytokines (IL-12) was also noted on splenic CD11c$^+$ DCs in mice treated with IDV. The capacity of IDV to modulate the immune response and enhance T cell activity through its effects on spelnic DCs is worth noting [29].

As mentioned previously, immunosuppressants and signaling or metabolic inhibitors also exhibit wide spectrum antimycotic activities. The topoisomerase I inhibitor camptothecin plus some of its derivatives [30] and the irreversible suicide inhibitor of ornithine decarboxylase eflornithine [31] have strong anti-*C. neoformans* activity. The sodium channel blocker amiodarone, conventionally used to treat arrhythmia, has potent anti-*S. cerevisiae* activity [32, 33]. Its effects are particularly pronounced in yeast mutants lacking key calcium transporter proteins. This is because unreplenished internal Ca^{2+} stores are depleted in a gradual but sustained manner [34]. Combination therapy with miconazole or fluconazole plus low doses of amiodarone greatly (>90%) reduces survival rate of *S. cerevisiae* and induces significant (>90%) *in vitro* killing of *C. albicans* and *C. neoformans* respectively [35].

Oligonucleotides

Targeting RNA with oligonucleotides for the purpose of disrupting their function is gaining momentum as a treatment approach for several forms of cancer and infectious diseases [36]. For instance, the anti-bcl-2 anti-sense messenger RNA construct Gentasense, along with other oligonucleotide preparations [37], is proving to be a potent drug in the treatment of acute myeloid leukemia. Vitravene™ is an antisense oligonucleotide that is proving to be effective against cytomegalovirus retinitis in AIDS patients intolerant, unresponsive or have contraindications to other treatment(s) of the infection [38]. The simple rules of base-pairing permit rational design, synthesis and testing of different oligonucleotides. Furthermore, features that influence oligonucleotide affinity to bind target RNA and its nuclease stability can be accommodated into the sequence design [39]. These two advantages are propelling RNA targeting by antisense oligonucleotides into the fore of anticancer and antiviral experimental therapies. This approach is also gaining some momentum in research and development of antifungal drugs. For, at any time point, complex eukaryotic fungal cells, contain in their intracellular environment large numbers of distinct RNA sequences involved in cell metabolism, housekeeping, viability and so on. Furthermore, recent evidence suggest that fungi like *C. albicans* can take up significant amounts of oligonucleotides in an energy-dependent manner where they remain stable for >12h [17]. Put together, these points provided for the development and testing of multiple oligonucleotides as potential antifungal agents. For example, a 19-mer with a *2'-O-methyl* backbone (19-mer2'-OMe) hairpin oligonucleotide was reported to inhibit *C. albicans* cell growth in culture at a pH of around 4.0, a pH that is easily tolerated in anatomic sites subject to candidiasis [17]. The oligonucleotide failed to inhibit the growth of mammalian COS-7 cells because uptake of the oligonucleotide by COS-7 cells in culture was 10-fold lower than that of *C. albicans* and because oligonucleotide stability inside COS-7 cells was minimal. This suggests that features such as oligonucleotide uptake by cells and stability of oligonucleotides within cells can vary depending on cell type, vis-à-vis fungal or mammalian. In other words, such features may provide a means for selective cell targeting.

It is now well-accepted that almost all RNA types (rRNA, RNase, P RNA, group I and group II introns and mRNAs with untranslated regulatory sequences) require secondary or tertiary folding to function properly [36, 40]. Generation of potential oligonucleotides by oligonucleotide directed misfolding of RNA (ODMiR), which uses short oligonucleotides to stabilize the inactive form of target RNA, has been described [37]. The oligonucleotides ^{L}(TACCTTTC) and $T^{L}CT^{L}AC^{L}GA^{L}CG^{L}GC^{L}C$ that target group I introns of *C. albicans* were generated by ODMiR and tested on *C. albicans* in culture. Both oligonucleotides were able to induce misfolds in group I introns and inhibit 50% of its splicing in different transcription mixtures [37]. Antisense repression of key genes in pathogenic fungi has been shown to alter their growth and reproduction [41]. For instance, serotype D yeast transformed with a plasmid containing the calcineurin A *(CNA1)* cDNA in an antisense orientation under the control of the inducible *GAL7* promoter demonstrated a temperature-sensitive phenotype only when grown on galactose, which was shown to be associated with decreased native *CNA1* transcript levels. It was also possible to modestly impair the growth of *C. neoformans* at 37°C by a 30bp antisense oligonucleotide targeting *CNA1* [41].

One of the potentially interesting anti-sense RNA molecules is the small (or short) interfering (or silencing) RNA (siRNA) [42]. siRNAs represent a class of double-stranded RNA molecules about 20-25 nucleotides in length. Through their ability to interfere with RNA metabolism, they can play a variety of roles in RNA expressing entities (cells and viruses). One of their most notable roles is their ability to interfere with the expression of select genes. Given their ability to essentially knock down any select gene, they are currently being tried as potential therapeutic agents against viral, bacterial, and fungal infections. For example, an anti-HIV siRNA-based treatment that knocks down specific HIV and host T cell genes (CCR5 viral co-receptor) was able to quash viral replication and prevent $CD4^+$ associated disease in infected humanized mice [43]. siRNA-based therapies are also being tried to treat fungal infections. For example, intranasal administration of siRNA preparations that specifically target the PI3K/Akt/mTOR inflammatory pathway in lung-derived DCs were recently shown to modify aspergillosis-related inflammation [44]. siRNA preps specifically targeting the STAT3/IDO anti-inflammatory pathway were able to modify immunity to aspergillosis [44].

Probiotic Therapy

Probiotic treatment involving the administration of living microorganisms in adequate quantities has been suspected of conferring some health benefits on the host since the days of *Eli Metchnikoff*. Lactic acid bacteria (LAB), bifidobacteria and some yeast species are currently used as probiotics against a wide array of infections and inflammatory diseases. Specific examples include *Lactobacilli* (*L. acidophilus*, *L. brevis*, *L. bulgaricus*, *L. casei*, *L. gasseri*, *L. paracasei*, *L. plantarum*, *L. rhamnosus*, *L. salivarius*, and *L. lactis*), *Streptococci* (*S. thermophilus*), *Bifidobacteria* (*B. bifidum*, *B. breve, B. infantis*, *B. lactis,* and *B. longum)*, and some yeasts (*S. cerevisiae*). Probiotics are thought to benefit the host by improving microbial balance that inhibits pathogens and toxin producing bacteria, alleviate chronic intestinal inflammatory diseases, prevent and treat pathogen-induced diarrhea, urogenital infections, and atopic diseases [45]. A study that has reviewed probiotic therapy literature published between 1966-1995 [46] has concluded that placebo-controlled studies have established that biotherapy can successfully prevent and/or treat antibiotic-associated diarrhea (*L. caseiGG*, *B. longum* with *L. acidophilus*, and *S. boulardii*), acute infantile diarrhea (*B. bifidum* with *S. thermophilus*), recurrent *Clostridium difficile* disease (*S. boulardii*), and various other diarrheal illnesses (*Enterococcus faecium* SF68, *L casei* GG, and *S boulardii*). The study also concluded that there exists ample evidence to support the contention that *L. acidophilus* probiotic therapy is effective at preventing vaginal candidiasis.

Criticisms of probiotic therapy have focused on sample size and degree of information masking in clinical trials conducted thus far, significant patient to patient benefit variations, cost effectiveness, and most importantly the generality of efficacy-gauging parameters employed [46]. For example, several studies and reviews have concluded that probiotic therapy can modulate anti-infection immunity [47-50]. In one study which used specific immune parameters however [51], out of 19 different biomarkers tested in subjects under academic examination stress, intake of milk fermented with yogurt cultures plus *L. casei* DN-114001 was only able to modulate the number of lymphocytes and that of $CD56^{+}$ (mostly NK) cells. Therefore, the ability of probiotic therapy to modulate immunity under stress conditions (infection or otherwise) is in doubt. Additionally, safety concerns especially in the immunocompromised and/or critically ill are yet to be resolved despite studies which have suggested that probiotic therapy is safe when given in oral [52] or topical form [46]. Cases of *lactobacillus* septicemia and allergic reactions in immunocompromised hosts have been reported [50, 53].

With regard to fungal infections, the majority of basic and clinical studies have focused on the potential of oral and topical use of different combinations of probiotics to prevent or reverse the dominance of pathogenic *Candida* species in the gastrointestinal and urogenital tracts [46, 54-58]. Probiotic therapy using a combination of *L. rhamnosus* GR-1 and *L. reuteri* RC-14 has proven effective at restoring and maintaining a normal vaginal microbiota through modulating host immunity, reducing pathogen ascension from the rectum, and interfering with colonization and survival of pathogens [47, 48]. Topical treatment with *Lactobacillus*–rich yogurt was shown to significantly reduce vaginal fungal burden in mice with estrogen-dependent vaginal candidiasis (EDVC) [56]. Furthermore, metronidazole-treated naïve mice developed persistent *C. albicans* vaginal colonization at levels significantly lower than that in untreated or metronidazole-treated EDVC mice suggesting that antibiotic therapy minimizes the benefits of probiotic therapy. A pilot, randomized, double-blind, placebo-controlled trial in human preterm neonates has demonstrated that *L. casei* GG administered in the first month of life significantly reduces enteric *Candida* colonization [55, 59]. During a 16-week, randomized, double-blind, placebo-controlled study with 136 elderly people consuming daily doses of 50g probiotic dairy products and 140 counterparts consuming daily doses of 50g cheese, the prevalence of *Candida* counts ($\geq$10 CFU/ml) decreased in the probiotic group from 30% to 21% and increased in the control group from 28% to 34% [55, 59]. Probiotic intervention reduced the risk of high yeast counts by 75% and the risk of hyposalivation by 56%.

It has been argued that the bacterial flora plays an important probiotic role in the prophylaxis of candidiasis by suppressing the growth of *Candida* species surviving on mucosal and cutaneous surfaces in immunocompromised hosts [54, 60]. Two commercially available isolates of *L. acidophilus* (NCFM and LA-1) were reported to protect immunedeficient bg/bg-nu/nu mice against candidiasis [60]. While use of *L. acidophilus* NCFM was able to prolong survival of adult and neonatal bg/bg-nu/nu mice and inhibit dissemination of candidiasis, *L. acidophilus* LA-1 was able to reduce the severity of mucosal candidiasis without significantly improving survival. The incidence of systemic candidiasis was significantly reduced and rates of survival were significantly improved in adult and neonatal athymic bg/bg-nu/nu mice by the presence of probiotic bacteria (*L. acidophilus*, *L. reuteri*, *L. casei* GG, or *B. animalis*) in the gastrointestinal tract [49]. Although no complete prevention of mucosal candidiasis was achieved, *B. animalis* was able to reduce incidence and severity of the disease. Furthermore, these probiotics were shown to modulate Ab- and cell-mediated immune responses to *C. albicans* [49].

LESSONS LEARNED

The task of managing fungal infections and lessening the harmful effects of chemotherapy is challenging to say the least. From the previous discussion it is clear that alternative therapies on the whole are prone to the development of resistance, have narrow spectrum of activity, and may associate with significant toxicity or harm to the host. Many of these therapies closely mimic conventional chemotherapy by targeting the pathogen (oligonucleotides, antineoplastics, biological blockers). Hence, they tend to associate with a similar set of drawbacks. Additionally, those that do not mimic chemotherapy *per se* (probiotics) are generalized food-supplements (rather than approved-drugs) with questionable efficacy and safety. So long as chemotherapy, or any type of therapy for that matter, continues to target the pathogen without engaging host immunity, problems will persist [2, 61]. Hence, engaging host immunity in direct and indirect ways should constitute part of the rationale in the search for therapies and control measures that complement chemotherapy or do away with it altogether. A more promising alternative approach to chemotherapy comes in the form of immune-based modalities and strategies [2, 61]. New insights into fungal immunity and pathology along with several technical advances in immunology and mycology are furnishing the essential tools to search for safe and effective immune-base antifungals. Hundreds of experimental fungal vaccines, monoclonal antibodies, cell transfer procedures, cytokine regimens, and other modalities have been developed and tested as agents to prevent and/or treat fungal infections. Before we get into all of that however, a relatively detailed introduction to fungal immunity is in order.

REFERENCES

[1] Abu Elteen K, Hamad M. (2005). Antifungal Compounds. In Kevin Kavanagh Editor. *Fungi: Biology and Applications* (pp.191-217). New York and London: Wiley.

[2] Abu Elteen K, Hamad M. (2007). Novel antifungal therapies. In Kevin Kavanagh Editor. *New Insights in Medical Mycology* (pp.69-98). Dordrecht: Springer Science and Business Media.

[3] Espinel-Ingroff A. (2009). Novel antifungal agents, targets or therapeutic strategies for the treatment of invasive fungal diseases: a review of the literature (2005-2009). *Rev. Iberoam. Micol.*, 26, 15-22.

[4] Bastidas RJ, Reedy JL, Morales-Johansson H, Heitman J, Cardenas ME. (2008). Signaling cascades as drug targets in model and pathogenic fungi. *Curr. Opin. Investig. Drugs*, 9, 856–864.

[5] Cruz, MC, Fox DS, Heitman J. (2001). Calcineurin is required for hyphal elongation during mating and haploid fruiting in *Cryptococcus neoformans*. *EMBO J.*, 20, 1020–1032.

[6] Bader T, Bodendorfer B, Schroppel K, Morschhauser J. (2003). Calcineurin is essential for virulence in *Candida albicans*. *Infect. Immun.*, 71, 5344–5354.

[7] Steinbach WJ, Schell WA, Blankenship JR, Onyewu C, Heitman J, Perfect JR. (2004). *In vitro* interactions between antifungals and immunosuppressants against *Aspergillus fumigatus*. *Antimicrob Agents Chemother*, 48, 1664–1669.

[8] Blankenship JR, Wormley FL, Boyce MK, Schell WA, Filler SG, Perfect JR, Heitman J. (2003). Calcineurin is essential for *Candida albicans* survival in serum and virulence. *Eukaryot Cell*, 2, 422–430.

[9] Uppuluri P, Nett J, Heitman J, Andes D. (2008). Synergistic effect of calcineurin inhibitors and fluconazole against *Candida albicans* biofilms. *Antimicrob. Agents Chemother*, 52, 1127–1132.

[10] Clipstone NA, Crabtree GR. (1993). Calcineurin is a key signaling enzyme in T lymphocyte activation and the target of the immunosuppressive drugs cyclosporin A and FK506. *Ann. NY Acad. Sci.*, 696, 20–30.

[11] Clipstone NA, Crabtree GR. (1992). Identification of calcineurin as a key signaling enzyme in T-lymphocyte activation. *Nature*, 357, 695–697.

[12] O'Keefe SJ, Tamura J, Kincaid RL, Tocci MJ, O'Neill EA. (1992). FK-506- and CsA-sensitive activation of the interleukin-2 promotner by calcineurin. *Nature*, 357, 692–694.

[13] Cardenas ME, Muir RS, Breuder T, Heitman J. (1995). Targets of immunophilin-immunosuppressant complexes are distinct highly conserved regions of calcineurin A. *EMBO J.*, 14, 2772–2783.

[14] Hemenway CS, Heitman J. (1999). Calcineurin. Structure, function, and inhibition. *Cell Biochem. Biophys.*, 30, 115–151.

[15] Cassone A, De Bernardis F, Santoni G. (2007). Anticandidal immunity and vaginitis: novel opportunities for immune intervention. *Infect. Immun.*, 75, 4675–4686.

[16] Denning DW. (2003). Echinocandin antifungal drugs. *Lancet*, 362, 1142–1151.

[17] Disney, M. D., Haidaris, C. G. and Turner, D. H.(2003). Uptake and antifungal activity of oligonucleotides in *Candida albicans*. Proc. Natl. Acad. Sci., 100:1530-1534.

[18] Gorlach, J. M., McDade, H. C., Perfect, J. R. and Cox, G. M. (2002). Antisense repression in *Cryptococcus neoformans* as a laboratory tool and potential antifungal strategy. *Microbiology*, 148:213–219.

[19] Cardenas, M. E., Cruz, M. C., Del Poeta, M., Chung, N., Perfect, J.R. and Heitman, J. (1999). Antifungal activities of antineoplastic agents: *Saccharomyces cerevisiae* as a model system to study drug action. *Clin. Microb. Rev*., 12:583-611.

[20] Del Poeta, M., Toffaletti, D. L., Rude, T. H., Dykstra, C. C., Heitman, J. and Perfect, J. R. (1999). Topoisomerase I is essential in *Cryptococcus neoformans*: role in pathobiology and as an antifungal target. *Genetics* 152:167-178.

[21] McCann, P. P., and Pegg, A. E. (1992). Ornithine decarboxylase as an enzyme target for therapy. *Pharmacol. Ther.* 54:195-215.

[22] Courchesne, W. E. (2002). Characterization of a novel, broad-based fungicidal activity of the antiarrhythmic drug amiodarone. *J. Pharmacol. Exp. Therap.,* 300:195-199.

[23] Courchesne, W. E. and Oztruk, S. (2003). Amiodarone induces a caffeine-inhibited, MID1-dependent rise in free cytoplasmic calcium in *Saccharomyces cerevisiae*. *Mol. Microbiol*., 47:223-234.

[24] Hatakka K, Ahola AJ, Yli-Knuuttila H, Richardson M, Poussa T, Meurman JH, Korpela R. (2007). Probiotics reduce the prevalence of oral candida in the elderly--a randomized controlled trial. *J. Dent Res.*, 86, 125-130.

[25] Manzoni P. (2007).Use of Lactobacillus casei subspecies Rhamnosus GG and gastrointestinal colonization by *Candida* species in preterm neonates. *J. Pediatr. Gastroenterol. Nutr.*, 45, S190-S194.

[26] Ibrahim AS, Gebermariam T, Fu Y, Lin L, Husseiny MI, French SW, Schwartz J, Skory CD, Edwards JE Jr, Spellberg BJ. (2007). The iron chelator deferasirox protects mice from mucormycosis through iron starvation. *J. Clin. Invest.*, 117, 2649-2657.

[27] Lee JH, Lee JY, Park JH, Jung HS, Kim JS, Kang SS, Kim YS, Han Y. (2007). Immunoregulatory activity by daucosterol, a beta-sitosterol glycoside, induces protective Th1 immune response against disseminated Candidiasis in mice. *Vaccine*, 25, 3834-3840.

[28] Gaziano R, Bozza S, Bellocchio S, Perruccio K, Montagnoli C, Pitzurra L, Salvatori G, Santis RD, Carminati P, Mantovani A, Romani L. (2004). Anti-*Aspergillus fumigatus* efficacy of pentraxin 3 alone and in combination with antifungals. *Antimicrob. Agents Chemother.*, 48, 4414–4421.

[29] Pericolini E, Cenci E, Gabrielli E, Perito S, Mosci P, Bistoni F, Vecchiarelli A. (2008). Indinavir influences biological function of dendritic cells and stimulates antifungal immunity. *J. Leukoc. Biol.*, 83, 1286-1294.

[30] Del Poeta M, Toffaletti DL, Rude TH, Dykstra CC, Heitman J, Perfect JR. (1999). Topoisomerase I is essential in *Cryptococcus neoformans*: role in pathobiology and as an antifungal target. *Genetics*, 152, 167-178.

[31] McCann PP, Pegg AE. (1992). Ornithine decarboxylase as an enzyme target for therapy. *Pharmacol. Ther.*, 54, 195-215.

[32] Courchesne WE. (2002). Characterization of a novel, broad-based fungicidal activity of the antiarrhythmic drug amiodarone. *J. Pharmacol. Exp. Therap.*, 300, 195-199.

[33] Courchesne WE, Oztruk S. (2003). Amiodarone induces a caffeine-inhibited, MID1-dependent rise in free cytoplasmic calcium in *Saccharomyces cerevisiae*. *Mol. Microbiol.*, 47, 223-234.

[34] Gupta AK, Cooper EA, Lynde CW. (2003). The efficacy and safety of terbinafine in children. *Dermatol. Clin.*, 21, 511-520.

[35] Thi L, Shaw D, Bird J. (2009). Warfarin potentiation: a review of the "FAB-4" significant drug interactions. *Consult Pharm.*, 24, :227-230.

[36] Disney, M. D., Matray, T., Gryaznov, S. M. and Turner, D. H. (2001). Recognition elements for 5' exon substrate binding to the *Candida albicans* group I intron. *Biochemistry,* 40:6520-6526.

[37] Childs JL, Disney MD. Turner DH. (2002). Oligonucleotide directed mis-folding of RNA inhibits *Candida albicans* group I intron splicing. *Proc. Natl. Acad. Sci.*, 99, 11091-11096.

[38] Galderisi U, Cascino A, Giordano A. (1999). Antisense oligonucleotides as therapeutic agents. *J. Cell Physiol.*, 181, 251-257.

[39] Freier SM, Altman KH. (1997). The ups and downs of nucleic acid duplex stability: structure-stability studies on chemically-modified DNA:RNA duplexes. *Proc. Natl. Acad. Sci.*, 25, 4429-4443.

[40] Testa SM, Gryaznov SM, Turner DH. (1999). *In vitro* suicide inhibition of self-splicing of a group I intron from *Pneumocystis carinii* by an N3' -> P5' phosphoramidate hexanucleotide. *Proc. Natl. Acad. Sci.*, 96, 2734-2739.

[41] Gorlach JM, McDade HC, Perfect JR, Cox GM. (2002). Antisense repression in *Cryptococcus neoformans* as a laboratory tool and potential antifungal strategy. *Microbiology*, 148, 213–219.

[42] Hamilton A, Baulcombe D. (1999). A species of small antisense RNA in posttranscriptional gene silencing in plants. *Science*, 286 (5441), 950–952.

[43] Kumar P, Ban HS, Kim SS, Wu H, Pearson T, Greiner DL, Laouar A, Yao J, Haridas V, Habiro K, Yang YG, Jeong JH, Lee KY, Kim YH, Kim SW, Peipp M, Fey GH, Manjunath N, Shultz LD, Lee SK, Shankar P. (2008). T cell-specific siRNA delivery suppresses HIV-1 infection in humanized mice. *Cell*, 134(4), 577-586.

[44] Bonifazi P, D'Angelo C, Zagarella S, Zelante T, Bozza S, De Luca A, Giovannini G, Moretti S, Iannitti RG, Fallarino F, Carvalho A, Cunha C, Bistoni F, Romani L. (2010). Intranasally delivered siRNA targeting PI3K/Akt/mTOR inflammatory pathways protects from aspergillosis. *Mucosal. Immunol.*, 2010, 3(2):193-205.

[45] Reid G, Jass J, Sebulsky T McCormick JK. (2003). Potential uses of probiotics in clinical practice. *Clin. Microbiol. Rev.*, 16, 658–672.

[46] Elmer GW, Surawicz CM, McFarland LV. (1996). Biotherapeutic agents. A neglected modality for the treatment and prevention of selected intestinal and vaginal infections. *JAMA*, 275, 870-876.

[47] Reid G. (2008). Probiotic Lactobacilli for urogenital health in women. *J. Clin. Gastroenterol.*, 42, S234-S236.

[48] Abad CL, Safdar N. (2009). The role of *Lactobacillus* probiotics in the treatment or prevention of urogenital infections--a systematic. *J. Chemother.*, 21, 243-252.

[49] Wagner RD, Pierson C, Warner T, Dohnalek M, Farmer J, Roberts L, Hilty M, Balish E. (1997). Biotherapeutic effects of probiotic bacteria on candidiasis in immunodeficient mice. *Infect. Immun.*, 65, 4165-4172.

[50] Prescott SL, Björkstén B. (2007). Probiotics for the prevention or treatment of allergic diseases. *J. Allergy Clin. Immunol.*, 120, 255-262.

[51] Marcos A, Wärnberg J, Nova E, Gómez S, Alvarez A, Alvarez R, Mateos JA, Cobo JM. (2004). The effect of milk fermented by yogurt cultures plus *Lactobacillus casei* DN-114001 on the immune response of subjects under academic examination stress. *Eur. J. Nutr.*, 43, 381-389.

[52] Joint FAO/WHO Working Group Report on Drafting Guidelines for the Evaluation of Probiotics in Food. April 30-May 1, 2002, London, Ontario, Canada.

[53] Besselink MG, van Santvoort HC, Buskens E, Boermeester MA, van Goor H, Timmerman HM, Nieuwenhuijs VB, Bollen TL, van Ramshorst B, Witteman BJ, Rosman C, Ploeg RJ, Brink MA, Schaapherder AF, Dejong CH, Wahab PJ, van Laarhoven CJ, van der Harst E, van Eijck CH, Cuesta MA, Akkermans LM, Gooszen HG. (2008). Probiotic prophylaxis in predicted severe acute pancreatitis: a randomised, double-blind, placebo-controlled trial. *Lancet*, 371, 651-659.

[54] Balish E, Wagner RD. (1998). Probiotic bacteria for prophylaxis and therapy of candidiasis. *Rev. Iberoam. Micol.*, 15, 261-264.

[55] Falagas ME, Betsi GI, Athanasiou S. (2006). Probiotics for prevention of recurrent vulvovaginal candidiasis: a review. *J. Antimicrob. Chemother.*, 58, 266-272.

[56] Hamad M, Muta'eb E, Abu-Shaqra Q, Fraij A, Abu-Elteen K, Yasin SR. (2006). Utility of the oestrogen-dependent vaginal candidosis murine model in evaluating the efficacy of various therapies against vaginal *Candida albicans* infection. *Mycoses*, 49, 104-108.

[57] Hatakka K, Ahola AJ, Yli-Knuuttila H, Richardson M, Poussa T, Meurman JH, Korpela R. (2007). Probiotics reduce the prevalence of oral candida in the elderly--a randomized controlled trial. *J. Dent. Res.*, 86, 125-130.

[58] Manzoni P, Mostert M, Leonessa ML, Priolo C, Farina D, Monetti C, Latino MA, Gomirato G. (2006). Oral supplementation with *Lactobacillus casei* subspecies rhamnosus prevents enteric colonization

by *Candida* species in preterm neonates: a randomized study. *Clin. Infect. Dis.*, 42, 1735-1742.

[59] Manzoni P. (2007). Use of *Lactobacillus casei* subspecies rhamnosus GG and gastrointestinal colonization by *Candida* species in preterm neonates. *J. Pediatr. Gastroenterol. Nutr.*, 45, S190-S194.

[60] Balish E. (2009). A URA3 null mutant of *Candida albicans* (CAI-4) causes oro-oesophageal and gastric candidiasis and is lethal for gnotobiotic, transgenic mice (Tgepsilon26) that are deficient in both natural killer and T cells. *J. Med. Microbiol.*, 58(Pt 3), 290-295.

[61] Hamad M. (2008). Antifungal immunotherapy and immunomodulation: a double-hitter approach to deal with invasive fungal infections. *Scand. J. Immunol.*, 67, 533–543.

Chapter 3

IMMUNITY TO FUNGI

During their evolutionary histories, vertebrates in general and mammals in particular have evolved elaborate defense mechanisms to ward off, fight, and clear fungal infections. This is well demonstrated by the fact that infections in immunocompetent hosts elicit innate and adaptive responses that collectively clear the infection and protect against subsequent infections. In contrast, immunocompromised hosts are susceptible to a whole host of opportunistic infections.

NO IMMUNITY NO PROTECTION

Evidence supporting the notion that defective, deficient, compromised, or aged immunity predisposes to fungal infections are overwhelming. The vast majority of opportunistic fungal infections occur in patients with compromised immunity (see table 3.1) such as those with cancer, AIDS, diabetes, organ transplants, and other underlying disease states [1-7]. Mice with autosomal or X-linked sever combined immunedeficiencies (SCIDs) and those with selective T cell (e.g. nude mutation *nu/nu* or *Foxn/nu* as it is now denoted) or granulocyte deficiencies are very susceptible to opportunistic fungal infections. Quantitative and qualitative defects of neutrophils, whether inherited or acquired, are associated with increased susceptibility to opportunistic fungal infections in animals and humans [8, 9]. Nicotinamide adenine dinucleotide phosphate (NADPH)-oxidase and myeloperoxidase deficiencies are associated with increased susceptibility to aspergillosis and pulmonary candidiasis [10]. Defects in proinflammatory T helper 1 (Th1) responses that tip the balance in favor of Th2 responses are associated with deleterious effects on the outcome of fungal infections [11]. Weakened immunity as a result of old age predispose to opportunistic fungal infections [12, 13]. Mice suffering from chronic granulomatous disease (CGD), a primary immunodeficiency marked by increased susceptibility to infection and inflammation, are highly susceptible to aspergillosis due to restricted activation of Th17 cells and unrestrained infection-induced inflammation [14].

Besides acquired and naturally-inherited immunodeficiencies, genetically-manipulated animal models have also demonstrated the essential role of various immune components, especially cell-mediated immunity (CMI), in the defense against various forms of mycosis. For example, epsilon 26 transgenic mice (Tgepsilon26) that lack the natural killer (NK) and T cell subsets are highly susceptible to alimentary tract colonization by wild-type *C. albicans*, avirulent URA3/URA3 null *C. albicans* mutants [15], and hyphal transcription factor signaling (efg1/efg1 and efg1/efg1 cph1/cph1) *C. albicans* mutants [16]. The URA3/URA3 (fungal pathogenesis gene) null *C. albicans* mutants can lethally colonize the alimentary tract, invade oral, esophageal, and gastric tissues, and evoke a granulocyte-dominated inflammatory response [14]. The efg1/efg1 or efg1/efg1/cph1/cph1 mutants can infect keratinized gastric tissues, increase the synthesis of cytokines (TNFα, IL-10 and IL-12) and chemokines (KC) and induce a granulocyte-dominated inflammatory response [16]. Germ-free BALB/c mice deficient for the IL-8 receptor homologue (IL-8Rh$^{-/-}$) are more susceptible to gastric and acute systemic candidiasis compared with wild-type counterparts [17]. Increased susceptibility in this case was attributed to slow influx of polymorphonuclear (PMN) cells into infected tissues and decreased representation of PMNs in peritoneal exudate cell (PEC) preparations. *C. albicans*-killing activity of PECs isolated from IL-8Rh$^{-/-}$ mice was lower than that exhibited by PECs isolated from of IL-8Rh$^{+/+}$ counterparts. Increased susceptibility to recurrent vulvovaginal candidiasis (RVVC) has recently been attributed to an early stop-codon mutation (Tyr238X) in the β-glucan receptor dectin-1 [18]. Mice deficient for CD192, a monocyte chemokine receptor, was reported to lead to defective inflammatory cell recruitment, increased IL-4 production and progressive histoplasmosis [19]. Mice lacking group V secretory phospholipase A2 (PLA2), an enzyme that hydrolyzes cell membrane phospholipids and releases fatty acids and lysophospholipids, experience increased fungal burden in the kidneys, liver, and spleen and increased mortality following infection with *C. albicans* [20].

Table 3.1. Defective immunity and the predisposition to opportunistic fungal infections

Opportunist infection	Immune impairment
Cryptococcosis	Defective CMI, drug-induced immunosuppression *
Aspergillosis	Neutropenia, drug-induced immunosuppression
Fusarium infections	Neutropenia, drug-induced immunosuppression, skin injuries, disrupted mucosa
Mucosal candidiasis	Defective CMI
Disseminated candidiasis	Neutropenia, defective CMI
Trichosporonosis	Neutropenia, skin injuries
Zygomycete infections	Neutropenia, drug-induced immunosuppression, diabetic ketoacidosis

* Corticosteroids and deferoxamine are among a group of widely used immunosuppressive drugs that associate with opportunistic fungal infections.

That being said, there are cases where certain forms of mycosis occur in healthy subjects. For instance, by challenging humans with live *C. albicans*, it has been demonstrated that while protection against vaginal candidiasis (VC) associates with non-inflammatory innate immunity, symptomatic infection correlates with high fungal burden and neutrophil infiltration of the vaginal lumen [21]. Based on these findings, it has been suggested that aggressive innate immunity rather than defective CMI is responsible for the development of symptomatic RVVC. Although mice deficient for TCR-$\alpha\beta^+$ (TCR-α knockouts) or TCR-$\gamma\delta^+$ (TCR-γ knockouts) T cells are highly susceptible to orogastric candidiasis, they are resistant to the disseminated and acute systemic forms of the infection [22]. Furthermore, it is well accepted that mucocutaneous fungal infections generally develop in people with no apparent immune defects. Finally, individuals with competent immunity are as likely to get dermatophytic infections as those with compromised immunity [23].

SETTING THE STAGE

There exist considerable temporal and spatial variations in the immune response profile against different forms of mycosis. Immunity against aspergillosis and pneumocystis depends on rapid pathogen recognition and deployment of effective innate responses followed by robust yet delayed adaptive responses. Immunity against *C. albicans* heavily depends on the type of infection being mucosal or systemic. In that, while resistance to *C. albicans* mucosal infections associates with Th1 responses, systemic infections typically associate with variable contributions of both Th1 and Th2 type responses. Additionally, while specific Ab responses and innate immunity components protect the host against invasive and disseminated candidiasis, mucocutaneous candidiasis is handled chiefly by CMI [24]. For dermatophytes, the role of CMI is to destroy the pathogen and render the host protected against re-infection. Resolution of dermatophytosis is generally associated with delayed type hypersensitivity (DTH). Immunity to various species of *Cryptococcus* is disparate enough to allow for differentiation between species based on differences in the immunological consequences that ensue following an infection. While *C. neoformans* mainly infects immunocompromised hosts, *C. gattii* tends to infect both immune-compromised and immunocompetent hosts. In general terms therefore, components of innate and acquired immunity converge to protect the host against fungal infections in spatial and temporal sequences that vary depending on the genus and/or species of the pathogen, its morphotype (mold, yeast, pseudohyphae, hyphae, mycelium etc.), and site of infection (localized, mucosal, systemic and so on) [25-27]. Such variations principally derive from differences in the sets of pathogenic determinants operative in different infectious agents and forms, the stage and site of infection, and the repertoire of expressed antigenic moieties and consequently the types of pathogen recognition and handling systems involved.

Like strain (and higher order-) based variations, phenotype (morphotype or simply type) switching, a phenomenon common to several fungal species, has considerable bearing on the quantitative and qualitative features of fungal immunity [28-31]. For it is involved in shaping the profile of morphotype-specific pathogenic determinants and virulence factors as well as the array of antigenic structures recognized by the host. Common examples of fungi that undergo phenotype switching include the dimorphic fungi *H. capsulatum, P. brasiliensis, C. immitis*, and *B. dermatitidis* that transform from saprobic filamentous molds to unicellular yeasts in the host. Other examples include the filamentous fungi *Aspergillus* species which transform into multicellular mycelia following inhalation as unicellular conidia and the yeast *Candida* species that grow into different phenotypes (yeast, blastospore, pseudohyphae, and hyphae). The dynamic changes that occur in *A. fumigatus* cell wall structure and synthesis significantly influence its ability to activate, suppress, or subvert host immunity [32]. This is well manifested in the differential ability of *A. fumigatus*-derived secreted and membrane-anchored proteins, glycolipids, and polysaccharides to induce Th1-mediated protective immunity in hematopoietic stem cell (HSC) transplant mice. It has been shown that host exposure to these fungal components leads to disparate immune consequences [32]. In that, while polysaccharides induce IL-10 production, secreted and membrane-anchored proteins and glycolipids activate Th2, Th1/Treg, and Th17 cells respectively. Furthermore, it has been reported that distinct intracellular pathways are activated following the recognition of different fungal morphotypes by distinct dendritic cell (DC) subsets. For example, inflammatory DCs are able to initiate the myeloid differentiation primary response gene (88) (MyD88)-dependent Th17/Th2 type immunity in response to *C. albicans* yeast infections. Tolerogenic DCs on the other hand respond to *C. albicans* hyphae by activating a toll-like receptor (TLR)/interleukin 1 receptor (IL-1R) domain-containing adaptor-inducing interferon-beta (IFN-β) (TRIF)-dependent Th1/Treg type immunity [33]. The plasticity of DC responses to different fungal antigens in this case was attributed to the involvement of the signal transducer and activator of transcription 3 (STAT3) that affects the activation of nuclear factor (NF)-κβ and indoleamine 2,3-dioxygenase (IDO). The expression of fungal antigens recognized by TLRs has been shown to significantly vary depending on *C. albicans* cell morphotype being yeast or hyphae [34].

As noted earlier, strain-based antigenic variations often replicate the effects of morphotype switching, vis-à-vis, generation of differential immunity against different strains of the same pathogen. In fact, along with variations in strain-specific (operative) virulence factors, antigenic differences and consequently differential immunity form the basis upon which differential susceptibility against different strains of the same pathogen can be understood. For example, although *C. neoformans* infections generally elicit robust Th1-mediated immunity, infection with *C. neoformans* H99 strain results in the generation of nonprotective Th2 type response and significant lung fungal burden. Interestingyl, IL-4 and IL-13 double knockout (IL-$4^{-/-}$/IL-$13^{-/-}$) mice challenged (by inhalation) with *C. neoformans* H99 strain were able to develop Th1/Th17, but not Th2, type immunity which associated with the prevention of pulmonary eosinophilia and airway goblet cell metaplasia, the elevation of serum IgE, and the switching from alternative to classical activation of macrophages [35]. The genetic background of the host also plays an important role in shaping the immune response against fungal infections. For example, varied immune responses to gastric candidiasis have been reported between two immunocompetent strains of mice that are equally susceptible to gastric candidiasis [36]. In that, while C57BL/6 mice respond to gastric candidiasis by upregulating the expression of some β-defensins (mBD1, mBD3, mBD4), chemokines (MIP-2, KC) and cytokines (IL-12 and TNF-α), BALB/c mice response is more specific and more subtle. Age is also worth considering as the robustness of immunity (adaptive and innate) wanes as the host grows older. For example, aged C57BL/6 mice intravenously infected with *C. albicans* hyphae experience low survival rates, high fungal burdens, decreased frequency of IFN-γ-producing $CD4^+$ T lymphocytes, and diminished *in vitro* ability of macrophages and splenocytes to respectively produce TNF-α and IFN-γ [6].

THE PARTICIPANTS

As stated earlier, various components of innate and acquired immunity come together to fight and clear fungal infections. In this context, appreaciating the relative importance of different immune components in protecting the host against various forms of mycosis is both relevant and contentious. Contentious because the working paradigm has been "*T cells vs the rest*". In other words, systemic and local adaptive CMI has long been regarded as the major player in defending against common fungal infections. In contrast, the role of antibody (Ab)-mediated immune responses has, until recently, been brushed aside as a negligible gig. Innate immunity has also been considered as passive, nonspecific, uninteresting, and uninformative aspect of fungal immunity.

T Cells

The historical emphasis on the role of adaptive CMI against fungal infections is not without devastating merits. T cells play a prominent protective role against systemic candidiasis, VC, chronic mucocutaneous candidiasis (CMC), aspergillosis, cryptococcosis, and many other fungal infections [8, 37-42]. Depletion of $CD4^+$ T cells is associated with increased susceptibility to *Pneumocystis pneumonia (P. pneumonia)* and other mycotic infections in rodents [41]. Differentiation of Th1 type responses is the determining factor of resistance to fungal infections [26]. Induction of Th1-mediated immunity by the secretion of IL-12, IFN-γ, and IL-6 confers significant protection against different forms of mycoses [43-45]. Positive lymphoproliferation characterized by overproduction of IFN-γ from cell cultures isolated from healthy individuals receiving cellular extracts of *A. fumigatus* or *A. fumigatus* antigens (the 88KD dipeptidase or the 90KD catalase) has been reported [44]. Increased levels of peripheral $CD4^+$ and $CD8^+$ memory T cells are detectable in patients infected with *P. brasiliensis* before and after chemotherapy [46]. In patients with relapsed infection, levels of IFN-γ are usually diminished, a finding that highlights the importance of IFN-γ in maintaining protective immunological memory against, at least some, fungal infections (e.g. *P. brasiliensis*) [46]. Polyfunctional $CD4^+$ lymphocytes, cells characterized by the ability to simultaneously produce IL-2, IFN-γ, and TNF-α, are detectable among peripheral blood lymphocytes (PBLs) in patients with coccidioidomycosis at a much higher frequency (12.5 times or a ratio of 137/11 per 400,000 events) than that in nonimmune patients [47]. $CD4^+CCR6^+$ T cells were reported to express IL-22, IL-17, and other Th1, Th2 or Th17 cytokines following stimulation of peripheral blood monocytes (PBMC) with heat-inactivated *C. albicans* yeast or hyphae [48]. It has been suggested that IL-17 produced by $CD3^+$ T cells in *H. capsulatum*-infected mice is essential for the induction of optimal inflammatory response and infection clearance [49]. It has also been demonstrated that mice lacking TCR-$\alpha\beta^+$ (TCR-α knockouts) or TCR-$\gamma\delta^+$ (TCR-γ knockouts) T cells are highly susceptible to orogastric candidiasis [22]. Additionally, there is evidence to suggest that whereas NK T cells promote Th1 immunity against *C. neoformans* infections, TCR$\gamma\delta^+$ T cells tend to suppress it [50]. In this context, it is worth noting that TCR-$\gamma\delta^+$ T lymphocytes play an important, though not fully appreciated, role in the defense against fungal infections; localized ones in particular [51, 52]. For example, TCR$\gamma\delta^+$ vaginal T lymphocytes (VTLs), which constitute an important part of the $CD3^+TCR^+CD90^+$ vaginal T cell population, exhibit a number of unique phenotypic, functional, and distribution features that enable them to provide tailor-made immune responses to localized (vaginal) infections [extensively reviewed in 52].

The Rest

The immense importance of CMI in defending against fungal infections notwithstanding, this paradigm has been challenged at several fronts [8, 37, 42, 43]. The ongoing appreciation of the role of DCs in recognizing fungal pathogens and initiating and orchestrating innate and acquired immunity to fungal infections is helping to reinstate innate immunity as an active and significant participant in fungal immunity. The heavy involvement of DCs in the immune response to fungal infections and their great potential as vaccines and *active* vaccine delivery systems qualifies them as pivotal players with pathogen-specific recognition and handling credentials (figure 3.1). The role of neutrophils and other phagocytes in mounting effector responses against a wide range of local and disseminated fungal infections is now well recognized [8, 42, 53-55]. Nothing demonstrates the importance of neutrophils in fungal immunity better than the fact that high rates of opportunistic fungal infections almost always associate with immunosuppression- or chemotherapy-induced neutropenia. Expression of innate immunity genes involved in recruitment, activation, and protection of neutrophils and monocytes (MNs) has been shown to significantly upregulate during the early phase of fungal infections [56, 57]. In addition to localized neutrophils and macrophages playing an important role in the defense against various fungal infections, clinical and experimental data suggest that different subsets of circulating monocytes are important as well. Recently, both $CD14^{+}CD16^{-}$ and $CD14^{+}CD16^{+}$ monocytes subsets isolated from healthy allogeneic HSC transplant donors were reported to be equally efficient at phagocytosing *A. fumigatus* conidia [32]. Using a cDNA microarray chip representing 42,421 genes, the expression of a large number of genes involved in cell function and survival significantly increased within 4-6 hours after incubation of human MNs infected with *C. albicans* [57]. Such genes included those of proinflammatory cytokines TNF-α, IL-1, IL-6, and leukemia inhibitory factor (LIF), chemokines IL-8 and macrophage inflammatory proteins (MIPs) 1, 3 and 4, MN chemoattractant protein-1 (MCAP1) and chemokine receptors CCR1, CCR5, CCR7, and CXCR5. The activity of MN viability-enhancing genes like BCL2-related protein, metallothioneins, CD71, and SOCS3 was also shown to upregulate within few hours of culture. Conversely, expression of genes adversely affecting MN function or viability (IL-15, IL-13Ra1, and CD14) was reported to downregulate during the 18 hour incubation period [57]. Upregulated expression of TLRs 2 and 4 was also reported following stimulation of human corneal epithelial cells (HCECs) with inactive *Fusarium solani* hyphae. Glucocorticoids (hydrocortisone) enhanced the expression of these TLRs on HCECs [56]. *H. capsulatum* infection in mice deficient for CCR2 (CD192), a receptor for MCAP1 on monocytes, was reported to lead to defective inflammatory cell recruitment, increased IL-4 production and progressive infection [19]. As neutralization of the CCR2 ligand CCL7 (but not the alternative ligand CCL2) was able to produce similar effects, it has been suggested that the ability of monocyte CCR2 to induce protective effects, which occurs through limiting IL-4 production, can be realized in the presence of CCL7.

Despite the lack of direct associations between defective Ab production/function and susceptibility to fungal infections, a growing list of supportive roles of Abs against several fungal infections is reviving the interest in Ab-mediated fungal immunity [58-66]. Systemic candidiasis (*C. albicans*), cryptoccocosis (*C. neoformans*) and other fungal infections often result in the production of opsonizing and complement-fixing Abs. There is evidence to suggest that anti-*Pneumocystis* Ab therapy is effective at preventing and treating *P. carinii* pneumonia (Pcp). Treatment with hyper-immune sera from mice immunized with *P. carinii* [67, 68] or with mAbs specific to *P. carinii* surface antigens [65, 69-71] resolved existing *P. carinii* infections in SCID mice and decreased hyperinflammatory reactions in immunoreconstituted mice. Complement fixation by the 4F11(G1) mAb was reported to be essential for optimal protection against infection with *P. carinii* and development of Pcp [72]. Infection by the melanin-producing *Fonsecaea pedrosoi*, the causative agent of chromoblastomycosis in humans, elicits production of anti-*F. pedrosoi* protective Abs [65]. Protective Abs can prevent biofilm formation by *C. neoformans* through interfering with capsular polysaccharide release from fungal cells [73]. Recovery from disseminated candidiasis in mice is associated with the presence of protective Abs against the molecular chaperone heat shock protein 90 (HSP90). Abs against pathogen-specific HSP90 epitopes and those against epitopes common to the pathogen and the host have been reported in patients recovering from systemic candidiasis [74, 75]. The expression, on phagocytes, of a unique immunoglobulin-γ3 (IgG3) receptor that is distinct from the common IgG (IgG1) crystallizable fragment receptor type γ (Fc-γR) has recently been shown to play a significant role in inducing protective Ab-mediated immunity against *C. neoformans* [76]. Through this unique receptor, IgG3 antibodies were able to efficiently opsonize *C . neoformans* in Fc-γR- and CD18-deficient cells and in the presence of blocking Abs to Fc-γR and complement receptors. Although pre-exposure to the IFN-γ-inducing *C. neoformans* strain H99γ, does elicit protective immunity against subsequent challenges, sensitized mice produce significant amounts of *C. neoformans*-specific Abs as compared with naïve mice [77]. That said, the importance of Ab-mediated immunity in protection against fungal infections remains contested, if not paradoxical. For example, as mentioned earlier, mice deficient for secretory IgM ($sIgM^{-/-}$) intraperitoneally-infected with *C. neoformans* strain 24067 can survive slightly longer than C57BL/6 x 129Sv control mice infected with the same pathogen

[78]. Naïve sIgM($^{-/-}$) mice generate higher levels of $CD5^+$ B-1 B cells, proinflammatory cytokines (IL-6, IL-1β, MIP-1 β, TNF-α, and IFN-γ), anti-inflammatory cytokines (IL-10 and IL-13), and GXM-specific IgG2a Abs. $CD5^+$ splenocytes from both mouse strains exhibit comparable fungicidal activities against *C. neoformans*. It seems therefore that this Ab deficiency renders the host more resistant to systemic cryptococcosis [78]. But in general terms, the fact remains that factors belonging to innate (mannose binding lectin [MBL], collectins, complement components) and humoral (Abs and complement cascades) immunity enhance antifungal innate defenses by facilitating fungal recognition, enabling complement activation and fixation, facilitating pathogen opsonization and neutralization and ultimately enhancing protective inflammation, [42, 43]. Although mice lacking C3 were reported to mount normal inflammatory responses, they were less capable of clearing *C. albicans* and *C. glabrata* infections [79].

Finally, For successful fungal commensalism and latency, immune responses against fungi need not be strong enough to eradicate the fungus nor weak enough to let the fungus run amok [8, 42]. To achieve this delicate balance between inflammation and tolerance, cooperation between various effectors and regulators deriving from the innate and adaptive arms of the immune system is needed (figure 3.2). One aspect of this coordinated process is the reciprocal relationship of neutrophil and T lymphocyte functions in protection against fungal infections [80, 81].

These aspects of fungal immunity go a long way in justifying why the "*T cells vs the rest*" paradigm is no longer valid and why and how it is being actively challenged. This point is very pertinent to the discussion here because taking aspects of fungal immunity besides adaptive CMI into account when thinking about strategies of and approaches to antifungal immunotherapy and immunomodulation is imperative.

THE PROCESS

Intact surfaces (epithelia and endothelia), microbial antagonism, physiological and biochemical barriers, and antimicrobial peptides (AMPs) collectively provide a preliminary passive line of defense that tends to ward off fungal infections. Once the pathogen enters the host through breached skin, mucosal lining injuries or inhalation, innate immunity cells sense the pathogen and mount an effector response to kill it or hold it in check. By doing so, innate immune responses prevent the pathogen from pathologically colonizing the tissue or disseminating to other tissues. Participants in this response include professional phagocytic cells; namely PMN cells (neutrophils), mononuclear (MN) cells (monocytes and macrophages) and DCs. Collectively, these cells recognize common fungal pathogen-associated molecular patterns (PAMPs), especially the cell wall-derived sugars, glycoproteins and glycolipids. Such fungal antigens or PAMPs are specifically recognized by different sets of pattern recognition receptors (PRRs) (table 3.1). Most notable are the TLR/IL-1R family of receptors (TLRs 2, 4, and 9 in particular), C-type lectin receptors (CLRs) dectin-1, dectin-2, DC-specific intercellular adhesion molecule-3-grabbing non-integrin (DC-SIGN or CD209), galectin, and the mannose receptor (MR). Other PRRs such as CR3 (CD11b/CD18) and other complement receptors, FcRs like the Fc-γR and the newly described FcR for IgG3, and MBL play an important role in innate fungal immunity as well. PRRs recognize a multitude of fungal antigens such as the cell wall-derived glucans (e.g. zymosan), mannose, mannans (polysaccharides), chitins and hundreds of other fungal sugars, proteins, glycoproteins and glycolipids. For example, glucuronoxylomannan (GXM) of *C. neoformans* is recognized by PAMP receptors TLR2, TLR4 and CD14 expressed on the surface of DCs and macrophages [82]. TLR2 and TLR4 on DCs and macrophages recognize a multitude of *A. fumigatus* cell wall-derived structures like zymosan and lipopolysaccharides. In brief, each and every fungal pathogen expresses (or produces) several (probably hundreds) antigens that can be recognized by one or more PRRs expressed on a variety of phagocytes within the host. This realization, not only highlights the importance of PRRs and innate immunity in general, but also suggests that subsequent interactions between the pathogen and the adaptive arm of host immunity are pre-conditioned by several (most probably distinct) PRR/PAMP interactions. Therefore, recognition of fungal PAMPs (mainly carbohydrate moieties) by phagocytes is a critical component of fungal immunity.

The Indispensable PRRs

In interacting with fungal pathogens like *C. albicans*, TLR2 may function as a homodimer or a heterodimer along with TLR1 or TLR6. It also combines with other PRRs in order to recognize fungal pathogens or initiate intracellular signaling cascades inside phagocytes to help fight the infection [34]. $TLR2^{-/-}$ mice intratracheally-infected with *P. brasiliensis*, were reported to develop mild pulmonary infection and decreased nitric oxide (NO) synthesis as compared with controls [83]. However, survival times and severity of pulmonary inflammatory reaction in TLR2$^{-/-}$ mice were similar to those observed in wild-type counterparts. Lung infiltrates in *P. brasiliensis*-infected TLR-2$^{-/-}$ mice consisted mainly of PMNs that control fungal loads; numbers of CD4^{+} and CD8^{+} T cell subsets were diminished, and the expansion of regulatory CD4^{+}CD25^{+}FoxP3^{+} T cells was impaired. Furthermore, increased production of KC, a CXC chemokine involved in neutrophils chemotaxis, TGF-β, IL-6, IL-23, and IL-17 was noticeable, perhaps suggestive of a skewed T cell response in favor of Th17 type response [83]. In a co-culture system consisting of *A. fumigatus* plus telomerase-immortalized corneal epithelial cells (THCE), it has been shown that THCE cells, which recognize the zymosan and lipopolysaccharide entities of *A. fumigatus* via TLR2 and TLR4 respectively, generated a signaling cascade that induced the production of IL-1β and IL-6 [84]. TLR2- and TLR4-mediated recognition of *C. albicans* and *A. fumigatus* antigens activated some members of the G protein-coupled protease-activated family of receptors and hence triggered distinct downstream signaling cascades that differentially influenced consequent immunity [85]. Although the contribution of TLR2 and TLR4 in the recognition of some fungal pathogens like *C. neoformans* remains contested [50], interaction of TLR9 with *C. neoformans*-derived DNA has been shown to mediate important MyD88-dependent intracellular signals.

Although TLRs are, by far, the main inducers of inflammation, the role of non-toll-like PRRs such as the CLRs as potential modulators of fungal immunity is being increasingly recognized [86-88]. CLRs have the potential to modulate inflammatory responses either by enhancing or inhibiting cytokine synthesis [86]. The dectins (dectin-1 in particular) and mincle, which is a CLR that is expressed predominantly on macrophages and plays a significant role in innate immunity to *C. albicans*, are cases in point. Mice lacking mincle show reduced levels of TNF-α production and high susceptibility to systemic candidiasis [89]. Among the most important CLRs is the β-glucan receptor dectin-1, which is expressed predominantly on the surface of cells of the myeloid lineage; mostly DCs and macrophages. Binding between dectin-1 and β-glucans initiates an intracellular signaling pathway that mediates cytokine production and other cellular responses [reviewed in 90]. Phagocytes (mainly macrophages and DCs) that express the dectin-1 exhibit potent anti-tumor and anti-microbial (viral, bacterial and fungal) activities owing to their ability to recognize β-glucans with a backbone of β -1,3/ β -1,6-linkages [91].

Table 3.1. A tentative list of signaling PRRS involved in fungal immunity

Receptor	Fungal ligand(s)	Adapter protein(s)	Location / cell type
Toll-like receptors (TLRs)			
TLR2	β-glucans (zymosan)	Mostly the MyD88-dependent pathway, occasionally the TIRAP (Mal)-, TRAM-, or TRIF-mediated pathways	Plasma membrane of monocytes, macrophages, and myeloid DCs
TLR4 (in conjunction with CD14, the LPS Binding Protein LBP, and MD	LPS, and single-stranded RNA		Plasma membrane of monocytes, macrophages, myeloid DCs, and mast cells
TLR9	Unmethylated CpG, oligodeoxynucleotid and DNA		Cell compartment monocytes, macrophages, and plasmacytoid DCs
C-type lectin receptors (CLRs)			
Dectin-1 (and Dectin-2)	β-glucans	Generally MyD88, Mal, or Src-Syk-CARD-9-Raf-1 (receptor-specific details are yet to be elucidated)	Phagocytes (macrophages and DCs)
DC-SIGN (human CD209)	Mannose type carbohydrates		Macrophages and myeloid and pre-plasmacytoid DCs
MB	Surface sugars with mannose termini		Phagocytes

In a recent study, use of a synthetic particulate β-glucan (p-β-glucan) was reported to significantly enhance the activity and phagocytosis of porcine alveolar macrophages (increased dectin-1, TLR4, TNF-α, and IL-12 production) and that of immature and mature DCs (inhibited IL-10 production) [91]. Although mucocutaneous fungal infections are rarely associated with defective immunity or immunodeficiency, RVVC has recently been linked to an early stop-codon mutation (Tyr238X) in the β-glucan receptor dectin-1 [18]. The mutation resulted in poor expression of defective dectin-1, which failed to mediate β-glucan binding. Following stimulation with β-glucan or *C. albicans in vitro*, the mutation resulted in defective production of IL-17, TNF, and IL-6 [18]. The mutation however did not affect fungal (*C. albicans*) phagocytosis or killing. Although dectin-1-knockout mice are more susceptible than wild-type counterparts to pneumocystis infections, both groups are equally susceptible to candidiasis suggesting that dectin-1 is required for immune responsiveness to some (but not necessarily all) fungal infections [92]. Additionally, disruption of dectin-1 does not result in impaired production of protective cytokines against cryptococcosis [50]. As part of the CLR family, galectin-3 participates in host immunity against microbial infections. Evaluation of the Th1/Th2 balance in C57BL/6 galectin-3-deficient (gal-$3^{-/-}$) mice infected with *P. brasiliensis* has revealed that, instead of the expected mixed type immune responsiveness to the infection, gal-$3^{-/-}$ mice were more susceptible to *P. brasiliensis*. Additionally, gal-$3^{-/-}$ mice exhibited a pattern of Th polarization that greatly favored Th2 type responses, which correlated with defective inflammatory and delayed type hypersensitivity (DTH) reactions, high IL-4 and GATA-3 expression and low NO production in infected organs [93].

Soluble pattern recognition proteins also participate in the handling of fungal antigens. For example, administration of pentraxin3 (PTX3), a multimeric pattern-recognition protein with potent anti-*Aspergillus* activity whose production is delayed in the case of CGD, following challenge with *A. fumigatus* was reported to restore antifungal resistance and limit the inflammatory response in mice with CGD [14]. This therapeutic effect of PTX3 was attributed to its ability to down-regulate IL-23 production by DCs and epithelial cells thereby permitting the expansion of inflammation-limiting Th1/Treg responses while limiting the expansion of IL-17A-producing IL-$23R^{+}$ $TCR\gamma\delta^{+}$ T cells [14].

Interestingly, besides mammals and vertebrates, other relatively simple organisms extensively use PRRs to recognize and handle fungal infections. For example, the nematode *Caenorhabditis elegans* (roundworm) uses the receptors CED-1 and C03F11.3 and their mammalian orthologue scavenger receptors SCARF1 and CD36 to recognize fungal β-glucans and mount immune responses against *C. neoformans* and *C. albicans* [94]. While CED-1 and C03F11.1 mediate antimicrobial peptide production which is essential for nematode survival, SCARF1 and CD36 mediate cytokine production and macrophage engagement with the pathogen.

Phagocytes in Action

Phagocytes kill fungi by oxidative and nonoxidative processes. Oxidative burst-dependent killing involves the NADPH oxidase- and the inducible NO synthase-mediated pathways. Therefore, NADPH-oxidase deficiency initiates the development of CGD by blocking the formation of reactive oxygen radicals and increasing host's susceptibility to aspergillosis [10]. The lysosomal hemoprotein myeloperoxidase that is present in abundance in the azurophilic granules of neutrophils and MNs represents another powerful oxygen-dependent mediator of fungal killing. Non-oxidative killing is mediated by collectins (pentraxin 3), defensins, neutrophil cationic peptides and numerous other AMPs that target and disrupt fungal cell membrane. In addition to their ability to kill microbes intracellularly following phagocytosis, neutrophils kill fungi extracellularly by degranulating antimicrobial proteins including the neutrophil extracellular traps (NETs), which was shown to contain a significant number (about 24) of associated proteins [95]. Many of these proteins localize to the cytoplasm in the unstimulated state. Release of the antimicrobial heterodimer calprotectin in response to *C. albicans* (and possibly other pathogens) represents the major antifungal component of NETs. This is based on the finding that calprotectin-deficient animals fail to clear *C. albicans* infections suggesting that absence of calprotectin from NETs compromises neutrophil antifungal activity [95]. Mice with impaired phagocyte function due to deficient phagocyte oxidase (Phox) plus NO synthase 2 (NOS2) or deficient production of reactive oxygen intermediates (ROI) and reactive nitrogen intermediates (RNI) are highly susceptible to infection by wild-type *C. albicans* and to hyphal signaling-defective mutants efg1/efg1 and efg1/efg1 cph1/cph1 of the pathogen [96]. This although peritoneal exudate cells isolated from NOS2$^{-/-}$, gp91phox$^{-/-}$/NOS2$^{-/-}$, or gp91phox$^{-/-}$ were as able to kill *C. albicans* cells *in vitro* just as those isolated from immunocompetent C57BL/6 mice [96]. Phagocytes can also restrict fungal growth and minimize infectivity through a whole host of mediators that deprive fungi of iron, inhibit dimorphism and block phenotype switching. It must be noted that although the heterogeneous population of tissue resident phagocytes (macrophages) has the potential to function as APCs, its main function is mostly restricted to phagocytosis and killing of fungi. Macrophages, in some cases, also participate in modulating immunity to fungi through the production of a number of cytokines in response to fungal infections [reviewed in 97].

Dendritic Cells: Movers and Shakers of Fungal Immunity

It is now recognized that DCs play the central role in initiating and orchestrating innate and acquired immunity against fungal infections (figure 3.1). In addition to the myeloid-derived mature DCs, immature DCs (iDCs) and plasmacytoid DCs (pDCs) are important in immunoprotection against fungi as well [8, 98]. For example, interaction of iDCs with the recombinant *A. fumigatus*-derived Aspf1 antigen results in upregulated expression of proinflammatory cytokines and augmented activation of NF-kβ [98]. The importance of DCs to immunity (fungal immunity in the present case) derives from several aspects of their biology and function:

(i) As described in table 3.1, DCs express a diverse set of PRRs that recognize and bind with a wide variety of fungal antigens expressed by most pathogenic fungi. The diverse repertoire of recognition and binding receptors expressed on DCs endows them with a pathogen-handling and -internalization plasticity unmatched by any other cell type. PRRs on DCs (TLRs, IL-1R, CR3, and MBLs) mediate distinct downstream signaling cascades that induce the synthesis of cytokines, AMPs and other signaling and effector molecules. The presence of conserved Toll/interleukin-1 receptor (TIR) domains in the cytosolic region of all TLR/IL-1R family of receptors on DCs allows them to generate signaling cascades similar to those that activate the transcription factor nuclear factor β (NFβ) and the stress-activated protein kinase family; both of which are involved in the activation and transcription of inflammatory and adaptive immune responses.

(ii) DCs are professional phagocytes; they internalize and process diverse sets of fungal peptides. Through different receptors and modes of phagocytosis, both human and mouse DCs can internalize *A. fumigatus, C. albicans, C. neoformans*, *H. capsulatum*, *Malassezia furfur*, *S. cerevisiae*, and others. DCs internalize yeasts and conidia predominantly by coiling phagocytosis, while hyphae internalization occurs by the more conventional zipper-type phagocytosis. Furthermore, recognition and internalization of unopsonized yeasts and conidia occurs through the engagement of DC-SIGN, dectin-1, CR3, and other cell wall sugar receptors. Therefore, the diverse set of PRRs expressed on DCs along with the capacity of DCs to cross-present internalized and exogenous fungal antigens released from dead phagocytes [99] enable them to decode and translate fungus-associated information into varied immune responses.

(iii) Signaling cascades initiated by the engagement between PRRs and PAMPs often recruit adapter proteins, most notably those associated with the MyD88 pathway. Besides the MyD88-dependent TLR-initiated signals however, CLRs and other non-toll-like PRRs generate distinct signaling cascades that activate and/or regulate immunity against fungi.

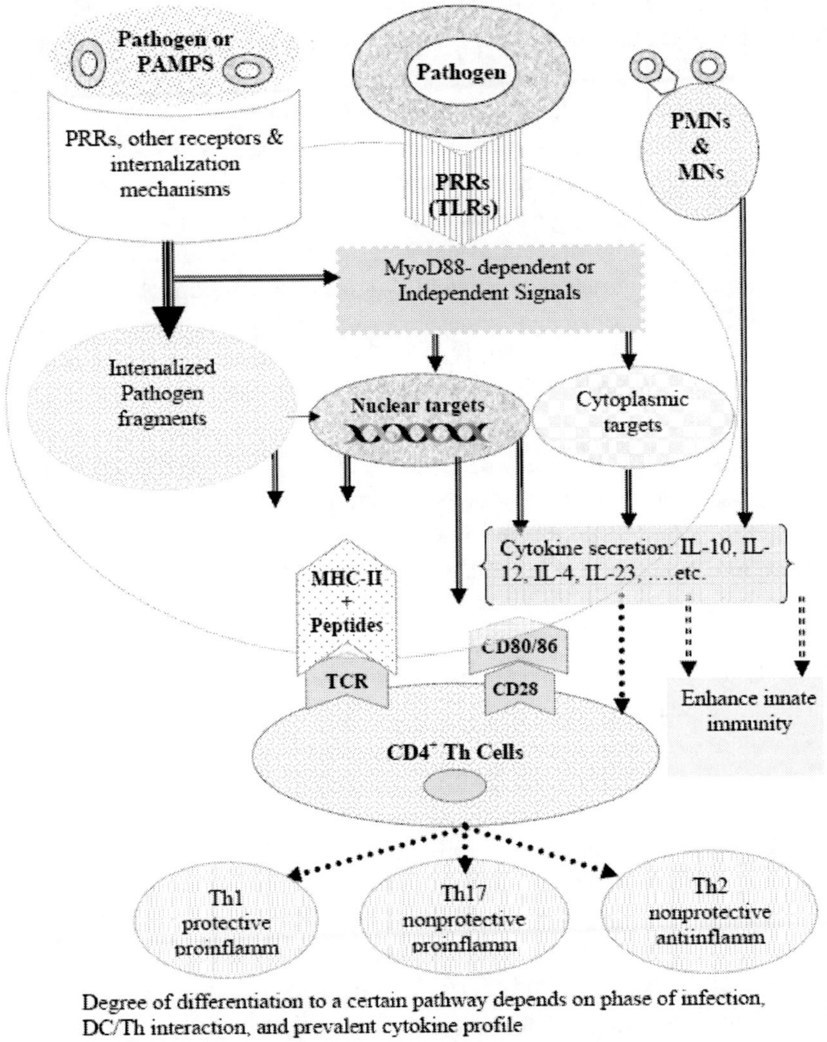

Figure 3.1. The central role of DCs in fungal immunity. Recognition and binding of fungal pathogen PAMPs by PRRs on DCs initiate both MyD88-dependent and –independent signaling cascades that collectively activate DCs , induce them to produce cytokines and AMPs, and enhance their ability to express MHC-II and T cell costimulatory molecule ligands. Phagocytosis of pathogens into DCs is followed by processing and presentation of fungal antigenic peptides to Th cells so as to initiate Th cell differentiation. These two main events endow DCs with the ability to initiate, orchestrate, and link diverse sets of innate and acquired responses against fungal pathogens.

For example, dectin-1-transduced signals involve a number of downstream signaling proteins such as Src/Syk kinases, CARD9 and Raf-1 [88, 90]. The ability of dectin-1 to recognize β-glucan-expressing pathogens and mediate signals to enhance immunity against them qualifies it as an important player in innate immunity against fungi [18, 88, 90-92].

Collectively, TLR/IL-1R-mediated MyD88-dependent signals and CLR-mediated Src/Syk/CARD9-dependent signals mobilize a diverse set of downstream signaling molecules and kinases. Most signals initiated by PRR-fungal pathogen interactions converge at the NF-κβ step. Activated NF-κβ induces DCs to produce cytokines and express ligands important to innate and/or adaptive immunity [100]. In other words, engagement of distinct receptors with distinct fungal morphotypes is translated by DCs into downstream signaling cascades that lead to upregulated production of cytokines like IL-12, IL-4, and IL-10, and upregulated expression of MHC-II and ligands for several T cell costimulatory molecules. CD80/CD86 (B7.1/B7.2) is one of the prime ligands expressed on DCs to bind with the T cell costimulatory molecules CD28 and CTLA-4 (CD152). It must be noted that upregulated expression of MHC-II on activated DCs restricts, to a large extent, their antigen presentation activities to $CD4^{+}$ T cells; hence their pivotal role in shaping the immune response. Furthermore, in what could be described as a positive feedback loop, cytokines produced by DCs activate DCs and amplify their capacity to detect, phagocytose and process fungal pathogens. IL-10 secreted by DCs in a MyD88-independent manner activates $CD4^{+}CD25^{+}$ T regulatory (Treg) cells, which are of prime importance in inducing and regulating antifungal resistance (figure 3.2) [reviewed in 8 and references therein]. Increased IL-10 production tends to downregulate production of the proinflammatory cytokine IFN-γ and consequently dampens antifungal CMI against chronic candidiasis and endemic mycoses.

(iv) Cytokines produced by DCs, and other phagocytes combined with the direct physical engagement between DCs and Th cells through concomitant ligand/costimulatory molecule binding and peptide-MHC-II/TCR interaction induces Th cell differentiation and cytokine production.

TH1/TH17 VS TH2

The differentiation of Th cells into Th1, Th2, or T17 pathways is largely determined based on the kinetics of peptide-MHC-II/TCR interaction and the prevailing cytokine profile influencing the process. The morphotype, and hence the specific fungal antigens, involved in the activation of DCs have some bearing on the differentiation pathway of naïve Th cells. For example, it has been reported that distinct intracellular pathways mediate the sensing of fungal conidia and hyphae by lung DCs *in vitro* [101]. Whereas the former translates into activation of Th1 protective responses, the later translates into activation of Th17 inflammatory responses. The consequences of Th differentiation into Th1, Th2, or T17 vary depending on the pathogen and site of infection. For the most part however, IL-12-driven differentiation of Th cells into Th1 and the consequent production of proinflammatory cytokines (IFN-γ, IL-6, IL-12 and TNF-β) is protective against most fungal infections, mucosal ones in particular [8, 42, 43, 102]. IFN-γ and other Th1 cytokines enhance the production and function of Abs (Abs) and enhance the recruitment and activity of innate immunity effector components. Additionally, cytokines released by phagocytes and Th cells engage and activate effector Tc cells.

Type 2 cytokines, IL-4 in particular, by acting to commit Th cells to the Th2 pathway at the expense of the Th1 pathway, dilute and counter Th1-mediated protective activity thus permitting fungal persistence and allergy. Elevated levels of IL-4 and other type 2 cytokines (IL-5, IL-10, IL-13) associate with diminished IFN-γ production, suppressed DTH responses, increased synthesis of nonprotective Abs (IgE, IgG4 and IgA), and eosinophilia [reviewed in references 42 and 102]. This profile positively correlates with fungal disease severity and poor prognosis. It must be noted however, that production of IL-4 or IL-5 is not always increased in patients with fungal infections (e.g. CMC infections) even if Th1 type cytokine production is defective [103].

IL-23-driven differentiation of Th cells into the Th17 pathway is believed to be a distinct lineage that is separate from the Th1 pathway. This is, of course, despite the close structural similarities between IL-12 and IL-23 and the fact that IL-23 functions through a receptor complex that consists of IL-12Rβ1 subunit plus components of the IL-23R chain. Like IL-12, IL-23 induces Th cells to produce proinflammatory cytokines (e.g. IFN-γ), however unlike IL-12, it induces Th cells to uniquely express IL-17. Th17 cells also produce IL-17F, IL-21, and IL-22 which, along with IL-17, play a significant immunological role during viral, bacterial, and fungal infections at different mucosal surfaces [104]. The activity of IL-17-producing T cells has been associated both with increased protection against microbial infections and excessive (injurious) inflammation. It has been suggested that IL-17 produced by $CD3^+$ T cells in *H. capsulatum*-infected mice is essential for the induction of optimal inflammatory response and pathogen clearance [49]. Additionally, defects in Th17 cell development and differentiation has been associated with increased susceptibility to recurrent pneumonia resulting from filamentous fungi and to mucocutaneous candidiasis in patients with primary immunodeficiencies. On the other hand, there is strong evidence to suggest that IL-17 is a negative regulator of Th1-mediated protective immunity and that it measurably impairs immune resistance and promotes inflammation [8, 105, 106]. Moreover, the activity of IL-17-producing T cells has been shown to associate with increased predisposition to various pathologies including autoimmunity [106]. Th17 responses against fungal infections (*C. albicans* and *A. fumigatus*) were reported to subvert neutrophil inflammatory responses, promote fungal virulence, and exacerbate inflammation and infection [8, 42, 106]. Based on these observations, it is likely that the IL-23/IL-17 pathway correlates far greater with severity and pathology of infectious diseases than with protection against disease [107, 108].

Immunotherapeutic measures to counter the nonprotective and inflammatory tendencies of Th2 and Th17 responses in hosts with defective or compromised immunity may prove beneficial. It has been suggested that inhibition of IL-17 production could lead to better modulation of the inflammatory response against *A. fumigatus* [109]. Additionally, the capacity of cytokine inhibitors (e.g. anti-IL-4 Abs) to block the differentiation of non-protective Th2 cells and enhance the differentiation of protective Th1 responses has been demonstrated [110].

INFLAMMATION VS TOLERANCE: A BALANCING ACT

In the rush to minimize tissue colonization and pathogen persistence, Th1 immunity recruits and activates effector immune components that clear the pathogen and cause significant inflammation. The activity of Th17, while dampening protective Th1 immunity, tips the balance in favor of further inflammation and tissue injury. Inversely, Th2 responses impair protective Th1 immunity by enhancing anti-inflammatory responses thus permitting the pathogen to colonize and persist within the host. Under normal circumstances, there seems to be some sort of a balancing act between proinflammatory and anti-inflammatory responses that ultimately leads to optimal immunity. However, the "Th1/Th17/Th2 alone" paradigm may not convincingly explain the exquisite and subtle balance between proinflammatory and anti-inflammatory tolerogenic responses in hosts with competent immunity. In other words, by only considering Th1, Th17, and Th2 responses acting on their own, the routine transition from the proinflammatory phase to the anti-inflammatory phase of the immune response would be rough and bumpy. This is particularly true given the massive and sudden changes in proinflammatory and anti-inflammatory cytokine concentrations and the minimal overlap between the two phases. Therefore, a new paradigm that could better explain the smooth generation of immune responses that are strong enough to fight and nearly clear infections without leading to pathologic inflammation and full tissue sterilization is needed (figure 3.2). It is worth mentioning here that full clearance of the pathogen within the timelines of the immune response is never desirable as it deprives the host of developing a level of tolerance sufficient to generate and maintain immunologic memory. Currently, it is postulated that the task of finely tuning and balancing protective (Th1) and nonprotective (Th17) proinflammatory responses on the one hand and nonprotective anti-inflammatory (Th2) responses on the other, falls upon T regulatory (Treg) cells [8, 42, 43, 72, 85]. Several subsets of the thymus-derived, naturally occurring Treg cells ($CD4^{+}CD25^{+}FoxP3^{+}$) and adaptively differentiated Tregs ($CD4^{+}CD25^{+}FoxP3^{-}$) secret sets of cytokines (IL-10, tumor growth factor-beta (TGF-β), and IL-4) that tend to keep Th1, Th17, and Th2 responses in check (figure 3.2) [24, 81, 103, 105, 107].

As discussed previously, IL-10 that is primarily produced by DCs and Treg cells in response to fungal mannans and other cell wall polysaccharides, negatively affects IFN-γ production, weakens CMI, and dampens Th1 responses against chronic candidiasis, severe forms of endemic mycoses, and aspergillosis in neutropenic patients [42]. IDO, the enzyme that mediates tryptophan (Trp) catabolism to N-formylkynurenine, can cause Trp depletion in target cells and halt their growth and activity [103]. It has been postulated [8] that during the early phase of fungal infections, IL-10 and CTLA-4, by acting on IDO, suppress the activity of recruited neutrophils to limit inflammation and tissue damage. In the late phase of the infection, IL-10 and TGF-β inhibit Th2 responses in order to limit pathogen persistence and allergy. Specialized DC subsets like the granulcocyte monocyte colony stimulating factor (GM-CSF)/IL-4-stimulated myeloid DCs and FLT3-ligand pDCs were reported to fulfill the requirements for Th1/Treg antifungal priming and tolerization [reviewed in 8]. Thymosin-α (Tα1), a modulator of human pDCs that functions through TLR9, was reported to affect these processes in DCs by activating the IDO-dependent pathway resulting in Treg development and tolerization [80]. This theme in fungal immunity, while leaving the door open for measured manipulations through DC and cytokine treatments, highlights some of the risks that could associate with such therapies. For instance, disturbing the Treg-initiated and maintained cytokine balance could easily tilt the immune response towards stronger inflammation and tissue damage or towards tolerance, pathogen persistence and allergy. Either of these two scenarios could lead to very adverse consequences. Vaccination with cell wall polysaccharides that induce IL-10 production could also replicate similar adverse effects.

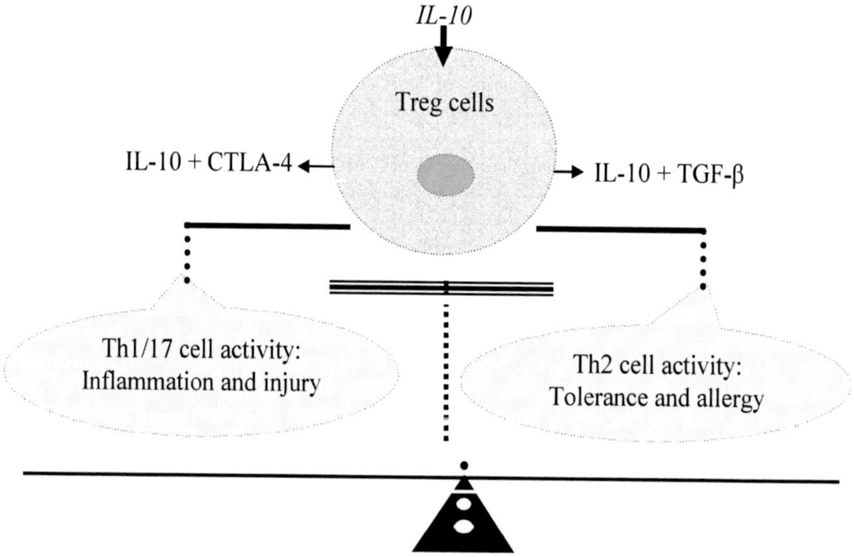

Figure 3.2. The balancing act of Treg cells. Balancing the activity of proinflammatory and anti-inflammatory cytokines is essential to minimize inflammation and permit pathogen tolerance. To achieve this goal, Treg cells produce cytokines (IL-10, TGF-β, etc.) that differentially activate, subvert, or suppress the activity of innate and acquired cellular components.

The Special Case of Dermatophytes

Dermatophytes are fungal molds that infect the skin and skin-derived keratinized structures (hair and nails). Dermatophytosis is somewhat unique among fungal infections in more than one respect. (i) Unlike common opportunistic fungal infections, infections caused by dermatophytes occur in healthy immunocompetent hosts just as prevalently as in patients with compromised immunity or with underlying disease states (e.g. atopic individuals, AIDS patients and so on) [23]. A human SCID case associated with an extensive *Trichophyton mentagrophytes (T. mentagrophytes)* skin infection has only recently been reported [111]. (ii) Infection-causing dermatophytes are not commensals of the host they infect; instead, they are usually caused by exogenous organisms. (iii) Some forms of dermatophytic infections usually present with inflammation (erythema, skin infiltration, pustule formation) such as those caused by zoophilic organisms. Other forms like tinea pedis (due to *T. rubrum*) tinea capitis (*T. tonsurans*) [112], and tinea imbricate (*T. concentricum*) [113] associate with little or no inflammation. Varied degrees of association between dermatophytosis and inflammation speak to different levels of neutrophil infiltration at the site of infection. (iv) Common dermatophytic infections (tinea pedis [soles], tinea capitis [scalp], tinea corporis [body], and tinea cruris [groin]) are superficial and almost never systemic or deep-seated. For dermatophytes to establish a skin infection (tinea) fungal propagules attach to the skin, germinate and overcome epidermal barriers. Consequently, host keratinocytes become activated and start to release of keratinases and other enzymes [114]. Disseminated forms of dermatophytosis involving internal organs are rare and often associate with defective immunity [115, 116]. (v) Dermatophytes tend to infect unusual targets (outer layers of the skin, hair, nails and the likes); they can also survive under stressful conditions. They, instead of relying on preached body surfaces to infect and colonize, can do the preaching on their own. Fungal cells largely responsible for dermatophytic infections (arthrospores; intercalary cells able to survive under harsh conditions) adhere to skin epidermis, secrete several tissue degrading-enzymes (proteases, metalloproteases and so on) [117] to help establish an infection. Collectivly, these aspects of dermatophytosis bear heavily on the way in which host immunity acts to protect against the disease. As a footnote to this issue, whether it is the difficulty in working with dermatophytosis or the lack of considerable interest in it; our level of understanding of the pathogenesis of and immunity to this group of infections remains superficial in comparison with that of common fungal infections.

Unlike the case in common fungal infections (candidiasis, aspergillosis, cryptococcosis, and so on), protection against dermatophytosis draws heavily on static as well as active components of the innate immune response. This is perhaps a suitable countermeasure to the ability of dermatophytes to attack intact healthy skin for the purpose of preaching it. Interaction of dermatophytes with unsaturated transferrin, activation of epidermal peptides, the inhibitory effects of fatty acids in sebum (e.g. undecylenic acid) and similar other processes play an active role in the defense against dermatophytosis. Although the mode of action of fatty acids is not well-understood, a chain length in the range of 7–13 carbon residues seems to be required for optimal *in vitro* antifungal activity [118]. Unsaturated transferrin, and to some extent lactoferrin, binds fungal cell membranes to physically inhibit their growth [119, 120]. Epidermally-derived antimicrobial peptides secreted by vertebrates exhibit both fungicidal and fungistatic activities against a wide variety of dermatophytes through interacting with the cell wall, cell membrane or the cytoplasm. Frog temporin and ranatuerin [121] and human cathelicidin [122] are epidermal peptides with potent antifungal (*T. rubrum* and *T. mentagrophytes*) activity. T cell-independent accelerated epidermal cell growth in mice and humans has also been shown to help in the clearance of pathogenic dermatophytes [121].

PMN cells, especially neutrophils, can infiltrate sites of dermatophytic infections (outer stratum corneum and hair follicle surroundings) and exact lethal hits against infecting fungi. In one study, it has been shown that human PMN can, in the course of 2 hours, kill up to 60% of dermatophyte germlings as compared with only 20% macrophage-mediated killing activity [23]. Neutrophils are recruited to the site of dermatophytosis by the production of epidermally (basal cell)-derived chemotactic factors like the leukotriene derivatives and by dermatophyte-derived cell wall antigens that tend to activate the alternate complement pathway [123]. In general terms, PMN cell-mediated killing is oxidative burst-dependent as evidenced by the fact that histidine and other inhibitors of free radicals like superoxide can inhibit dermatophyte killing [124, 125]. Phagocyte-mediated non-oxidative killing of dermatophytes is yet to be established [23].

The significant role of neutrophils in protection against dermatophytosis notwithstanding, evidence suggests that immunity against a number of human dermatophytic infections especially those that do not associate with inflammation (e.g. infections caused by anthropophilic fungi) is largely independent of neutrophil activity. For example, infection of glabrous skin in humans shows a clear lack of cellular infiltration [23, 126]. Additionally, the capacity of mammalian hosts to mount immune responses characteristic of secondary rather than primary immune responses to previously encountered dermatophytes suggests that dermatophytosis can lead to the induction of immunologic memory. These two aspects suggest that T cell immunity is involved in the defense against some, if not all, forms of dermatophytosis. Keratinophilic dermatophytes have been reported to elicit epidermal DC-orchestrated T cell-mediate immunity in mammalian hosts. Such epidermal

DCs bind dermatophyte-derived antigens via the CLR DC–SIGN [127]. Processed antigens are presented by DCs to local T cells or T cells residing within peripheral lymph nodes. In a mouse model of primary *T. quinckeanum* infection, polyclonal responsiveness of lymphocytes isolated from draining lymph nodes to the lectin mitogens concanavaline A (ConA) and phytohemaglutinin (PHA) was shown to be suppressed during infection peak period (day 7) as compared with that at day 30 (infection resolution period) post infection or that with monoclonal responsiveness to *T. quinckeanum*–derived antigens [128]. Furthermore, polyclonal responsiveness of lymphocytes isolated from mice with a secondary *T. quinckeanum* infection was significantly higher than that observed during the primary infection. Once again, monoclonal responsiveness in this case was more pronounced than polyclonal responsiveness especially at infection peak periods. Further analysis has revealed that cells expressing the suppressor phenotype Thy-1^+ Ly-2.2^+ ($CD90^+$ $CD8\alpha^+$) were responsible for inhibiting lymphocyte proliferation while cells expressing the helper phenotype $CD90^+$ $CD8\alpha^-$ were essential for the responsiveness of lymphocytes [128]. Transfer of the later, but not the former, cell population from immunized mice into naïve mice protected recipients against dermatophytosis. Interestingly, unlike the case of *Candida*- or *Aspergillus*-derived antigens that induce APCs like DCs to upregulate the expression of ligands for T cell co-stimulatory molecules [8, 42], dermatophytes tend to downregulate the expression of molecules like CD50 and CD80 [23].

Epidermal keratinocytes, not only function as effective physical barriers to dermatophytes, they also secret important immune mediators including proinflammatory cytokines, chemokines, and AMPs [129]. Human keratinocytes, when co-cultured with *T. mentagrophytes*, produce a number of cytokines such as IL-8 and TNF [130]. Co-culture of the keratinocyte cell line PHK16–0b with *T. mentagrophytes* upregulated the expression of genes encoding IL-1, IL-2, IL-4, IL-6, IL-13, IL-15, IL-16, and IFN-γ, while that with *T. tonsurans* induced the release of IL-8 and IL-16 and to some extent IL-1 [131]. Interestingly, *T. mentagrophytes*, human pathogenic dermatophytes that cause severe inflammation, elicit the release of many different cytokines as well. Macrophages interacting with *T. rubrum* conidia or hyphae can also produce TNF-α and IL-10 but not IL-12 or NO. These findings notwithstanding, the ability of host cells (epidermal or otherwise) present in the vicinity of infection to produce stimulatory and regulatory cytokines *in vivo* is yet to be investigated.

The exact role of T cell immunity in general and effector T cell immunity in particular and the underlying cellular and molecular mechanisms governing its anti-dermatophytic activity remains poorly understood. A number of dermatophyte-derived antigens like cell wall-derived glycopeptides, the HSP-60 family [132], metalloproteinases, and subtilases [133] can stimulate adaptive (B- and T cell-mediated) immunity and hence closely correlate with T cell activation and host resistance. On the other hand, some dermatophyte antigens can interfere with host adaptive immunity. For example, *Trichophyton*-derived antigens containing TQ-1 reactive epitopes were reported to increase the susceptibility of Balb/C mice to dermatophyte infection by blocking T cell-mediated immunity [134, 135]. Some oligosaccharides derived from dermatophyte cell wall glycolproteins can also disrupt the activation of both T and B lymphocyte. During acute dermatophytosis, a number of effector cells (lymphocytes and other cell types) are usually detectable in the area of the infection [136]. Such epidermal cell infiltrates include Leu2a$^+$ (CD8α^+) T helper cells [136, 137], CD8$\alpha\beta^+$ T cells, HLA-DR$^+$ cells, and Langerhans cells [23]. Recent evidence suggests that cellular defense mechanisms play an important role in clearing dermatophyte skin infections (tinea) [114].

AVENUES FOR IMMUNE-BASED INTERVENTION

Based on our current understanding of fungal immunity (figures 3.1 and 3.2), two distinct classes of immune-based antifungal interventions can be identified (see table 6.1). The first pertains to the wide array of agents and strategies that target the host to modulate and enhance its immunity to fungal infections, hence the term host-targeting immunomodulation (HTI). Under which, comes vaccines (native, recombinant, synthetic, antigen-pulsed DCs, etc.), cytokines, immunostimulatory Abs and peptides, as well as cell transfer (phagocytes, NK cells, and sensitized T cells) procedures. This approach helps to shift the focus from countering pathogen colonization and infectivity to enhancing anti-pathogen host immunity. Complementary (or alternative) to HTI is a set of immunological agents that target and kill fungal pathogens, inhibit their growth or hinder their mobility and infectivity, hence the name pathogen-targeting immunotherapy (PTI). This includes blocking, opsonizing and neutralizing Abs (whole or fragmentary, monoclonal or polyclonal, naked or conjugated with radioactive or cytocidal agents) and AMPs (natural or synthetic, native or modified). Like chemotherapy, PTI, by definition, focuses on the pathogen and does little to modulate or enhance host immunity. Each of these two general approaches has advantages and disadvantages, they sometimes overlap, and each presents powerful tools to combat fungal infections. The focus of HTI and PTI being different, vis-à-vis host vs pathogen, entails differences between these two categories in terms of spectrum of activity, ability to induce resistance, and potential to precipitate toxic side effects as will be discussed at some length in chapter 6. Modalities comprising HTI have, for the most part, broad spectrum of activity, reduced toxicity and minimal risk of inducing resistance. On the negative side however, issues like inflammation and allergic reactions, accelerated vaccine-induced pathogen strain replacement, and the need for competent immunity are troubling. PTI on the other hand acts independent of host immunostatus and its narrow spectrum of activity can be compensated for by the relative ease with which pathogen-specific Abs can be designed or by the generation of pan-fungi mAbs. However, serious side effects and the likelihood of resistance development are two major drawbacks.

REFERENCES

[1] Pfaller MA, Diekema DJ. (2007). Epidemiology of invasive candidiasis: a persistent public health problem. *Clin. Microbiol. Rev.*, 20, 133–163.

[2] De Pauw BE. (2006). Increasing fungal infections in the intensive care unit. *Surg Infect (Larchmt)*, 7 (Suppl. 2), S93-S96.

[3] Enoch DA, Ludlam HA, Brown NM. (2006). Invasive fungal infections: a review of epidemiology and management options. *J. Med. Microbiol.*, 55, 809-818.

[4] Hamad M. (2008). Antifungal immunotherapy and immunomodulation: a double-hitter approach to deal with invasive fungal infections. *Scand. J. Immunol.*, 67, 533–543.

[5] Fidel P, Barousse M, Espinosa T, Ficarra M, Sturtevant J, Martin DH, Quayle AJ, Dunlap K. (2004). An intravaginal live *Candida* challenge in humans leads to new hypotheses for the immunopathogenesis of vulvovaginal candidiasis. *Infect. Immun.*, 72, 2939–2946.

[6] Murciano C, Villamón E, Yáñez A, O'Connor JE, Gozalbo D, Gil ML. (2006). Impaired immune response to *Candida albicans* in aged mice. *J. Med. Microbiol.*, 55, 1649-56.

[7] Quezada G, Koshkina NV, Zweidler-McKay P, Zhou Z, Kontoyiannis DP, Kleinerman ES. (2008). Intranasal granulocyte-macrophage colony-

stimulating factor reduces the *Aspergillus* burden in an immunosuppressed murine model of pulmonary aspergillosis. *Antimicrob. Agents Chemother*, 52, 716–718.

[8] Romani L. (2007). Immunity to Fungi. In Kevin Kavanagh Editor. *New Insights in Medical Mycology* (pp. 1-19). Dordrecht: Springer Science and Business Media,

[9] Bennett JE. (2009). The changing face of febrile neutropenia-from monotherapy to moulds to mucositis. Management of mycoses in neutropenic patients: a brief history, 1960-2008. *J. Antimicrob. Chemother.*, 63 (Suppl 1), i23-i26.

[10] Segal B, Leto T, Gallin J, Malech H, Holland S. (2000). Genetic, biochemical, and clinical features of chronic granulomatous disease. *Medicine (Baltimore)*, 79, 170–200.

[11] Jancovic D, Liu Z, Gause WC. (2001). Th1- and Th2-cell commitment during infectious diseases: asymmetry in divergent pathways. *Trends Immunol.*, 22, 450–457.

[12] Simitsopoulou M, Roilides E, Likartsis C, Ioannidis J, Orfanou A, Paliogianni F, Walsh TJ. (2007). Expression of immunomodulatory genes in human monocytes induced by voriconazole in the presence of *Aspergillus fumigatus*. *Antimicrob. Agents Chemother.*, 51, 1048–1054.

[13] Laube S. (2004). Skin infections and ageing. *Ageing Res. Rev.*, 3, 69-89.

[14] D'Angelo C, De Luca A, Zelante T, Bonifazi P, Moretti S, Giovannini G, Iannitti RG, Zagarella S, Bozza S, Campo S, Salvatori G, Romani L. (2009). Exogenous pentraxin 3 restores antifungal resistance and restrains inflammation in murine chronic granulomatous disease. *J. Immunol.*, 183(7), 4609-4618.

[15] Balish E. (2009). A URA3 null mutant of *Candida albicans* (CAI-4) causes oro-oesophageal and gastric candidiasis and is lethal for gnotobiotic, transgenic mice (Tgepsilon26) that are deficient in both natural killer and T cells. *J. Med. Microbiol.*, 58(Pt 3), 290-295.

[16] Westwater C, Balish E, Warner TF, Nicholas PJ, Paulling EE, Schofield DA. (2007). Susceptibility of gnotobiotic transgenic mice (Tgepsilon26) with combined deficiencies in natural killer cells and T cells to wild-type and hyphal signalling-defective mutants of *Candida albicans*. *J. Med. Microbiol.*, 56(Pt 9), 1138-1144.

[17] Balish E, Wagner RD, Vazquez-Torres A, Jones-Carson J, Pierson C, Warner T. (1999). Mucosal and systemic candidiasis in IL-8Rh-/- BALB/c mice. *J. Leukoc. Biol.*, 66(1), 144-150.

[18] Ferwerda B, Ferwerda G, Plantinga TS, Willment JA, van Spriel AB, Venselaar H, Elbers CC, Johnson MD, Cambi A, Huysamen C, Jacobs L, Jansen T, Verheijen K, Masthoff L, Morré SA, Vriend G, Williams DL, Perfect JR, Joosten LA, Wijmenga C, van der Meer JW, Adema GJ, Kullberg BJ, Brown GD, Netea MG. (2009). Human dectin-1 deficiency and mucocutaneous fungal infections. *N. Engl. J. Med.*, 361(18), 1760-1767.

[19] Szymczak WA, Deepe GS Jr. (2009). The CCL7-CCL2-CCR2 axis regulates IL-4 production in lungs and fungal immunity. *J. Immunol.*, 183(3), 1964-1974.

[20] Balestrieri B, Maekawa A, Xing W, Gelb MH, Katz HR, Arm JP. (2009). Group V secretory phospholipase A2 modulates phagosome maturation and regulates the innate immune response against *Candida albicans*. *J. Immunol.*, 182(8), 4891-4898.

[21] Fidel PL Jr. (2007). History and update on host defense against vaginal candidiasis. *Am. J. Reprod. Immunol.*, 57(1), 2-12.

[22] Jones-Carson J, Vazquez-Torres A, Warner T, Balish E. (2000). Disparate requirement for T cells in resistance to mucosal and acute systemic candidiasis. *Infect. Immun.*, 68(4), 2363-2365.

[23] Hay RJ. (2007). Immune responses to dermatophytoses. In Kevin Kavanagh Editor. *New Insights in Medical Mycology* (pp.227-240). Dordrecht: Springer Science and Business Media.

[24] Richardson M, Rautemaa R. (2009). How the host fights against *Candida* infections. *Front Biosci.*, 14, 4363-4375.

[25] Shoham S, Levitz ML. (2005). The immune response to fungal infections. *British Journal of Hematology*, 129, 569-82.

[26] Matthews RC, Burnie JP. (2004). Recombinant antibodies: a natural partner in combinatorial antifungal therapy. *Vaccine*, 22, 865-71.

[27] Blanco JL, Garcia ME. (2008). Immune response to fungal infections. *Vet. Immunol. Immunopathol.*, 125, 47-70.

[28] Jain N, Cook E, Xess I, Hasan F, Fries D, Fries BC. (2009). Isolation and characterization of senescent *Cryptococcus neoformans* and implications for phenotypic switching and pathogenesis in chronic cryptococcosis. *Eukaryot Cell*, 8, 858-866.

[29] Jain N, Li L, Hsueh YP, Guerrero A, Heitman J, Goldman DL, Fries BC. (2009). Loss of allergen 1 confers a hypervirulent phenotype that resembles mucoid switch variants of *Cryptococcus neoformans*. *Infect. Immun.*, 77, 128-140.

[30] Pietrella D, Fries B, Lupo P, Bistoni F, Casadevall A, Vecchiarelli A. (2003). Phenotypic switching of *Cryptococcus neoformans* can influence the outcome of the human immune response. *Cell Microbiol.*, 5, 513-522.

[31] Fries BC, Taborda CP, Serfass E, Casadevall A. (2001). Phenotypic switching of *Cryptococcus neoformans* occurs in vivo and influences the outcome of infection. *J. Clin. Invest.*, 108, 1639-1648.

[32] Bozza S, Clavaud C, Giovannini G, Fontaine T, Beauvais A, Sarfati J, D'Angelo C, Perruccio K, Bonifazi P, Zagarella S, Moretti S, Bistoni F, Latgé JP, Romani L. (2009). Immune sensing of *Aspergillus fumigatus* proteins, glycolipids, and polysaccharides and the impact on Th immunity and vaccination. *J. Immunol.*, 183, 2407-2414.

[33] Bonifazi P, Zelante T, D'Angelo C, De Luca A, Moretti S, Bozza S, Perruccio K, Iannitti RG, Giovannini G, Volpi C, Fallarino F, Puccetti P, Romani L. (2009). Balancing inflammation and tolerance *in vivo* through dendritic cells by the commensal *Candida albicans*. *Mucosal Immunol*, 2(4), 362-374.

[34] Gil ML, Gozalbo D. (2009). Role of Toll-like receptors in systemic *Candida albicans* infections. *Front Biosc.*, 14, 570-582.

[35] Zhang Y, Wang F, Tompkins KC, McNamara A, Jain AV, Moore BB, Toews GB, Huffnagle GB, Olszewski MA. (2009). Robust Th1 and Th17 immunity supports pulmonary clearance but cannot prevent systemic dissemination of highly virulent *Cryptococcus neoformans* H99. *Am. J. Pathol.*, 175(6), 2489-2500.

[36] Schofield DA, Westwater C, Balish E. (2005). Divergent chemokine, cytokine and beta-defensin responses to gastric candidiasis in immunocompetent C57BL/6 and BALB/c mice. *J. Med. Microbiol.*, 54(Pt 1), 87-92.

[37] Fidel PL. Immunity to *Candida*. Oral Disease 2002; 8:69-75.

[38] Lindell DM, Moore TA, McDonald RA, Toews GB, Huffnagle GB. (2005). Generation of antifungal effector $CD8^+$ T cells in the absence of $CD4^+$ T cells during *Cryptococcus neoformans* infection. *J. Immunol.*, 174, 7920-7928.

[39] Harmsen AG, Stankiewicz M. (1990). Requirements for $CD4^+$ cells in resistance to *Pneumocystis carinii* pneumonia in mice. *J. Exp. Med.*, 172, 937-945.

[40] Phair J, Munoz A, Detels R, Kaslow R, Rinaldo C, Saah A. (1990). The risk of *Pneumocystis carinii* pneumonia among men infected with

human immunodeficiency virus type 1.Multicenter AIDA Cohort Study Group. *N. Engl. J. Med.*, 322, 161-165.
[41] Thullen TD, Ashbaugh AD, Daly KR, Linke MJ, Steele PE, Walzer PD. (2003). New rat model of *Pneumocystis* pneumonia induced by the anti-$CD4^+$ T-lymphocyte antibodies. *Infect. Immun.*, 71, 6292-6297.
[42] Romani L. (2004). Immunity to fungal infections. *Nat. Rev. Immunol.*, 4, 1–23.
[43] Romani L. (2002). Immunology of invasive candidiasis. In Calderone RA Editor. *Candida* and *Candidiasis* (pp. 223-241). Washington DC: ASM Press.
[44] Hebart H, Bollinger C, Fisch P, Sarfati J, Meisner C, Baur M, Loeffler J, Monod M, Latgé JP, Einsele H. (2002). Analysis of T-cell responses to *Aspergillus fumigatus* antigens in healthy individuals and patients with hematologic malignancies. *Blood*, 100, 4521-4528.
[45] Cenci E, Mencacci A, Fe d'Ostiani C, Del Sero G, Mosci P, Montagnoli C, Bacci A, Romani L. (1998). Cytokine- and T helper-dependent lung mucosal immunity in mice with invasive pulmonary aspergillosis. *J. Infect. Dis.*, 178, 1750-1760.
[46] Bozzi A, Reis BS, Goulart MI, Pereira MC, Pedroso EP, Goes AM. (2007). Analysis of memory T cells in the human paracoccidioidomycosis before and during chemotherapy treatment. *Immunol. Lett.*, 114, 23-30.
[47] Nesbit L, Johnson SM, Pappagianis D, Ampel NM. (2010). Polyfunctional T lymphocytes are in the peripheral blood of donors naturally immune to coccidioidomycosis and are not induced by dendritic cells. *Infect. Immun.*, 78(1), 309-315.
[48] Liu Y, Yang B, Zhou M, Li L, Zhou H, Zhang J, Chen H, Wu C. (2009). Memory IL-22-producing CD4+ T cells specific for *Candida albicans* are present in humans. *Eur. J. Immunol.*, 39(6), 1472-1479.
[49] Deepe GS Jr, Gibbons RS. (2009). Interleukins 17 and 23 influence the host response to *Histoplasma capsulatum*. *J. Infect. Dis.*, 200(1), 142-51.
[50] Kawakami K. (2009). Recognition mechanism of pathogen-associated molecular patterns and role of innate immune lymphocytes in fungal infection. *Rinsho Byori*, 57(8), 779-785.
[51] Poggi A, Catellani S, Musso A, Zocchi MR. (2009). Gammadelta T lymphocytes producing IFNgamma and IL-17 in response to *Candida albicans* or mycobacterial antigens: possible implications for acute and chronic inflammation. *Curr. Med. Chem.*, 16(35), 4743-4749.

[52] Hamad M. (2008). The case for extrathymic development of vaginal T lymphocytes. *J. Reproductive Immunology*, 77, 109-116.

[53] Vora S, Purimetla N, Brummer E, Stevens DA. (1998). Activity of voriconazole, a new triazole, combined with neutrophils on monocytes against *Candida albicans*: Effect of granulocyte colony-stimulating factor and granulocyte-monocyte colony stimulating factor. *Antimicrob Agents Chemother*, 42, 907-910.

[54] Roilides E, Holmes A, Blake C, Pizzo PA, Walsh TJ. (1993). Impairment of neutrophil fungicidal activity against *Aspergillus fumigatus* in HIV-infected children. *J. Infect. Dis.*, 167, 905-911.

[55] Razonable RR, Henault M, Lee LN, Laethem C, Johnston PA, Watson HL, Paya CV. (2005). Secretion of pro-inflammatory cytokines and chemokines during amphotericin B exposure is mediated by co-activation of toll-like receptors 1 and 2. *Antimicrob. Agents Chemother.*, 49, 1617-1621.

[56] Jin X, Qin Q, Tu L, Zhou X, Lin Y, Qu J. (2007). Toll-like receptors (TLRs) expression and function in response to inactivate hyphae of *Fusarium solani* in immortalized human corneal epithelial cells. *Mol. Vis.*, 13, 1953-1961.

[57] Kim HS, Choi EH, Khan J, Roilides E, Francesconi A, Kasai M, Sein T, Schaufele RL, Sakurai K, Gue Son C, Greer BT, Chanock S, Lyman CA, Walsh TJ. (2005). Expression of genes encoding innate host defense molecules in normal human monocytes in response to *Candida albicans*. *Infect. Immun.*, 73, 3714–3724.

[58] Targan SR, Hanauer SB, van Deventer SJ, Mayer L, Present DH, Braakman T, DeWoody KL, Schaible TF, Rutgeerts PJ. (1997). A short-term study of chimeric monoclonal antibody cA2 to tumor necrosis factor alpha for Crohn's disease cA2 Study group. *N. Engl. J. Med.*, 337, 1029-1035.

[59] Casadevall A. (1995). Antibody immunity and invasive fungal infections. *Infect. Immun.*, 63, 4211-4218.

[60] Rivera J, Casadevall A. (2005). Mouse genetic background is a major determinant of isotype-related differences for antibody-mediated protective efficacy against *Cryptococcus neoformans*. *J. Immunol.*, 174, 8017-8026.

[61] Han Y, Cutler JE. (1995). Antibody response that protects against disseminated candidiasis. *Infect. Immun.*, 63, 2714-2719.

[62] Matthews R, Hodgets S, Burnie J. (1995). Preliminary assessment to of a human recombinant antibody fragment to hsp90 in murine invasive candidiasis. *J. Infect. Dis.*, 171, 1668-1671.

[63] Dromer F, Charreire J, Contrepois A, Carbon C, Yeni P. (1987). Protection of mice against experimental cryptococcosis by anti-*Cryptococcus neoformans* monoclonal antibody. *Infect. Immun.*, 55, 749-752.

[64] Mukherjee J, Pirofski IA, Scharf MD, Casadevall A. (1994). Antibody mediated protection in mice with lethal intracerebral *Cryptococcus neoforman* infection. *Proc. Natl. Acad. Sci. USA*, 90, 3636-3640.

[65] Daniela S. Alviano, Anderson J. Franzen, Luiz R. Travassos, Carla Holandino, Sonia Rozental, Regina Ejzemberg, Celuta S. Alviano, and Marcio L. Rodrigues. (2004) Melanin from *Fonsecaea pedrosoi* induces production of human antifungal antibodies and enhances the antimicrobial efficacy of phagocytes. *Infect. Immun.*, 72, 229–237.

[66] Pachl J, Svoboda P, Jacobs F, Vandewoude K, van der Hoven B, Spronk P, Masterson G, Malbrain M, Aoun M, Garbino J, Takala J, Drgona L, Burnie J, Matthews R. (2006). A randomized, blinded, multicenter trial of lipid-associated amphotericin B alone versus in combination with an antibody-based inhibitor of heat shock protein 90 in patients with invasive candidiasis. *Clin. Infect Dis.*, 42, 1404-1413.

[67] Roths JB, Sidman CL. (1992). Both immunity and hyperresponsiveness to *Pneumocystis carinii* result from transfer of $CD4^+$ but not $CD8^+$ T cells into severe combined immunodeficiency mice. *J. Clin. Investig.*, 90, 673–678.

[68] Roths JB, Sidman CL. (1993). Single and combined humoral and cell-mediated immunotherapy of *Pneumocystis carinii* pneumonia in immunodeficient SCID mice. *Infect. Immun.*, 61, 1641–1649.

[69] Gigliotti F, Haidaris CG, Wright TW, Harmsen AG. (2002). Passive intranasal monoclonal antibody prophylaxis against murine *Pneumocystis carinii* pneumonia. *Infect. Immun.*, 70, 1069–1074.

[70] Lee LH, Gigliotti F, Wright TW, Simpson-Haidaris PJ, Weinberg GA, Haidaris CG. (2000). Molecular characterization of KEX1, a kexin-like protease in mouse *Pneumocystis carinii*. *Gene*, 242, 141–150.

[71] Wells J, Gigliotti F, Simpson-Haidaris PJ, Haidaris CG. (2004). Epitope mapping of a protective monoclonal antibody against *Pneumocystis carinii* with shared reactivity to *Streptococcus pneumoniae* surface antigen PspA. *Infect. Immun.*, 72, 1548–1556.

[72] Wells J, Haidaris CG, Wright TW, Gigliotti F. (2006). Complement and Fc function are required for optimal antibody prophylaxis against *Pneumocystis carinii* pneumonia. *Infect. Immun.*, 74, 390–393.
[73] Martinez LR, Casadevall A. (2005). Specific antibody can prevent fungal biofilm formation and this effect correlates with protective efficacy. *Infect. Immun.*, 73, 6350-6362.
[74] Matthews RC. (1992). *Candida albicans* HSP90: Link between protective and auto immunity. *J. Med. Microbiol.*, 36, 367-370.
[75] Matthews RC. (1994). Pathogenicity determinants of *Candida albicans*: Potential targets for immunotherapy. *Microbiology*, 104, 1505-1511.
[76] Saylor CA, Dadachova E, Casadevall A. (2010). Murine IgG1 and IgG3 isotype switch variants promote phagocytosis of *Cryptococcus neoformans* through different receptors. *J. Immunol.*, 184(1), 336-343.
[77] Young M, Macias S, Thomas D, Wormley FL Jr. (2009). A proteomic-based approach for the identification of immunodominant *Cryptococcus neoformans* proteins. *Proteomics*, 9(9), 2578-2588.
[78] Subramaniam KS, Datta K, Marks MS, Pirofski LA. (2010). Improved survival of mice deficient in secretory immunoglobulin M following systemic infection with *Cryptococcus neoformans*. *Infect. Immun.*, 78(1), 441-452.
[79] Tsoni SV, Kerrigan AM, Marakalala MJ, Srinivasan N, Duffield M, Taylor PR, Botto M, Steele C, Brown GD. (2009). Complement C3 plays an essential role in the control of opportunistic fungal infections. *Infect. Immun.*, 77(9), 3679-3685.
[80] Montagnoli C, Perruccio K, Bozza S, Bonifazi P, Zelante T, De Luca A, Moretti S, D'Angelo C, Bistoni F, Martelli M, Aversa F, Velardi A, Romani L. (2008). Provision of antifungal immunity and concomitant alloantigen tolerization by conditioned dendritic cells in experimental hematopoietic transplantation. *Blood Cells Mol. Dis.*, 40, 55-62.
[81] Romani L, Puccetti P. (2008). Immune regulation and tolerance to fungi in the lungs and skin. *Chem. Immunol. Allergy*, 94, 124-137.
[82] Yauch LE, Mansour MK, Shoham S, Rottman JB, Levitz SM. (2004). Involvement of CD14, toll-like receptors 2 and 4, and MyD88 in the host response to the fungal pathogen *Cryptococcus neoformans in vivo*. *Infect. Immun.*, 72, 5373-5382.
[83] Loures FV, Pina A, Felonato M, Calich VL. (2009). TLR2 is a negative regulator of Th17 cells and tissue pathology in a pulmonary model of fungal infection. *J. Immunol.*, 183(2), 1279-1290.

[84] Guo H, Wu X. (2009). Innate responses of corneal epithelial cells against *Aspergillus fumigatus* challenge. *FEMS Immunol. Med. Microbiol.*, 56(1), 88-93.

[85] Moretti S, Bellocchio S, Bonifazi P, Bozza S, Zelante T, Bistoni F, Romani L. (2008). The contribution of PARs to inflammation and immunity to fungi. *Mucosal. Immunol.*, 1(2), 156-168.

[86] Ferwerda G, Netea MG, Joosten LA, van der Meer JW, Romani L, Kullberg BJ. (2010). The role of Toll-like receptors and C-type lectins for vaccination against *Candida albicans*. *Vaccine*, 28(3), 614-622.

[87] Willment JA, Brown JD. (2008). C-type lectin receptors in antifungal immunity. *Trends in Microbiology*, 16(1), 27-32.

[88] Gross O, Gewies A, Finger K, Schäfer M, Sparwasser T, Peschel C, Förster I, Ruland J. (2006). Card9 controls a non-TLR signalling pathway for innate anti-fungal immunity. *Nature*. 442(7103), 651-656.

[89] Wells CA, Salvage-Jones JA, Li X, Hitchens K, Butcher S, Murray RZ, Beckhouse AG, Lo YL, Manzanero S, Cobbold C, Schroder K, Ma B, Orr S, Stewart L, Lebus D, Sobieszczuk P, Hume DA, Stow J, Blanchard H, Ashman RB. (2008). The macrophage-inducible C-type lectin, mincle, is an essential component of the innate immune response to *Candida albicans*. *J. Immunol.*, 180, 7404-7413.

[90] Reid DM, Gow NA, Brown GD. (2009). Pattern recognition: recent insights from Dectin-1. *Curr. Opin. Immunol.*, 21(1), 30-37.

[91] Chaung HC, Huang TC, Yu JH, Wu ML, Chung WB. (2009). Immunomodulatory effects of beta-glucans on porcine alveolar macrophages and bone marrow haematopoietic cell-derived dendritic cells. *Vet. Immunol. Immunopathol.*, 131(3-4), 147-157.

[92] Saijo S, Fujikado N, Furuta T, Chung SH, Kotaki H, Seki K, Sudo K, Akira S, Adachi Y, Ohno N, Kinjo T, Nakamura K, Kawakami K, Iwakura Y. (2007). Dectin-1 is required for host defense against *Pneumocystis carinii* but not against *Candida albicans*. *Nat. Immunol.*, 8, 39-46.

[93] Ruas LP, Bernardes ES, Fermino ML, de Oliveira LL, Hsu DK, Liu FT, Chammas R, Roque-Barreira MC. (2009). Lack of galectin-3 drives response to *Paracoccidioides brasiliensis* toward a Th2-biased immunity. *PLoS One*, 4(2), e4519.

[94] Means TK, Mylonakis E, Tampakakis E, Colvin RA, Seung E, Puckett L, Tai MF, Stewart CR, Pukkila-Worley R, Hickman SE, Moore KJ, Calderwood SB, Hacohen N, Luster AD, El Khoury J. (2009). Evolutionarily conserved recognition and innate immunity to fungal

pathogens by the scavenger receptors SCARF1 and CD36. *J. Exp. Med.*, 206(3), 637-53.

[95] Urban CF, Ermert D, Schmid M, Abu-Abed U, Goosmann C, Nacken W, Brinkmann V, Jungblut PR, Zychlinsky A. (2009). Neutrophil extracellular traps contain calprotectin, a cytosolic protein complex involved in host defense against *Candida albicans*. *PLoS Pathog*, 5(10): e1000639.

[96] Balish E, Warner TF, Nicholas PJ, Paulling EE, Westwater C, Schofield DA. (2005). Susceptibility of germfree phagocyte oxidase- and nitric oxide synthase 2-deficient mice, defective in the production of reactive metabolites of both oxygen and nitrogen, to mucosal and systemic candidiasis of endogenous origin. *Infect. Immun.*, 73(3), 1313-1320.

[97] Vázquez-Torres A, Balish E. (1997). Macrophages in resistance to candidiasis. *Microbiol. Mol. Biol. Rev.*, 61, 170-192.

[98] Ok M, Latgé JP, Baeuerlein C, Ebel F, Mezger M, Topp M, Kurzai O, Killian D, Kapp M, Grigoleit GU, Sennefelder H, Arroyo J, Einsele H, Loeffler J. (2009). Immune responses of human immature dendritic cells can be modulated by the recombinant *Aspergillus fumigatus* antigen Aspf1. *Clin. Vaccine Immunol.*, 16(10):1485-92.

[99] Lin JS, Yang CW, Wang DW, Wu-Hsieh BA. (2005). Dendritic cells cross-present exogenous fungal antigens to stimulate a protective CD8 T cell response in infection by *Histoplasma capsulatum*. *J. Immunol.*, 174, 6282–6291.

[100] Kawai T, Akira S. (2005). Toll-like receptor downstream signaling. *Arthritis Res. Ther.*, 7, 12-19.

[101] Bonifazi P, D'Angelo C, Zagarella S, Zelante T, Bozza S, De Luca A, Giovannini G, Moretti S, Iannitti RG, Fallarino F, Carvalho A, Cunha C, Bistoni F, Romani L. (2010). Intranasally delivered siRNA targeting PI3K/Akt/mTOR inflammatory pathways protects from aspergillosis. *Mucosal. Immunol.*, 2010, 3(2):193-205.

[102] Romani L, Kaufmann SH. (1998). Immunity to fungi: editorial overview. *Res. Immunol.*, 149, 277-281.

[103] Lilic D, Gravenor I, Robson N, Lammas DA, Drysdale P, Calvert JE, Cant AJ, Abinun M. (2003). Deregulated production of protective cytokines in response to *Candida albicans* infection in patients with chronic mucocutaneous candidiasis. *Infect. Immun.*, 71, 5690-5699.

[104] Khader SA, Gaffen SL, Kolls JK. (2009). Th17 cells at the crossroads of innate and adaptive immunity against infectious diseases at the mucosa. *Mucosal. Immunol.*, 2(5), 403-411.

[105] Curtis MM, Way SS. (2009). Interleukin-17 in host defense against bacterial, mycobacterial and fungal pathogens. *Immunology*, 126, 177-85.

[106] Zelante T, De Luca A, D'Angelo C, Moretti S, Romani L. (2009). IL-17/Th17 in anti-fungal immunity: what's new? *Eur. J. Immunol.*, 39(3), 645-648.

[107] Stumhofer JS, Silver J, Hunter CA. (2007). Negative regulation of Th17 responses. *Semin. Immunol.*, 19, 394-399.

[108] Hunter CA. (2005). New IL-12-family members: IL-23 and IL-27, cytokines with divergent functions. *Nat. Rev. Immunol.*, 5, 521-531.

[109] Chai LY, van de Veerdonk F, Marijnissen RJ, Cheng SC, Khoo AL, Hectors M, Lagrou K, Vonk AG, Maertens J, Joosten LA, Kullberg BJ, Netea MG. (2010). Anti-*Aspergillus* human host defense relies on type 1 T helper (Th1), rather than type 17 T helper (Th17), cellular immunity. *Immunology,* [Epub ahead of print].

[110] Roilides E, Dignani MC, Anaissie EJ, Rex JH. (1998). The role of immune-reconstitution in the management of refractory opportunistic fungal infections. *Med. Mycol.*, 36, 12–25.

[111] Jiménez-Puya R, Vázquez-Bayo C, Rodriguez-Bujaldón A, Gómez García F, Moreno-Giménez JC. (2009). Extensive tinea in a patient with severe combined immunodeficiency. *Pediatr. Dermatol.*, 26(2), 213-214.

[112] Elewski B. (1999). Treatment of tinea capitis: beyond griseofulvin. *J. Am. Acad. Dermatol.*, 40, S27–S30.

[113] Serjeantson S, Lawrence G. (1977). Autosomal recessive inheritance of susceptibility to tinea imbricate. *Lancet*, 1, 13–15.

[114] Brasch J. (2009). Current knowledge of host response in human tinea. *Mycoses*, [Epub ahead of print].

[115] Allen DE, Snyderman R, Meadows L, Pinnell SR. (1977). Generalized *Microsporum audoninii* infection and depressed cellular immunity associated with a missing plasma factor required for lymphocyte blastogenesis. *Am. J. Med.*, 63, 991–1000.

[116] Liautaud B, Marill FG. (1984). Dermatophytic disease. Recent Algerian observations. *Bull Soc. Fr. Pathol. Exotique*, 77, 637–648.

[117] Brouta F, Descamps F, Monod M, Vermout S, Losson B, Mignon B. (2002) Secreted metalloprotease gene family of *Microsporum canis*. *Infect. Immun.*, 70, 5676–5683.

[118] Abraham A, Mohapatra LN, Kandhari KC. (1975). The effects of some hair oils and unsaturated fatty acids on experimentally induced dermatophytosis. *Dermatologica*, 151, 144–149.

[119] King RD, Khan HA, Foye JC, Greenberg JH, Jones HE. (1975). Transferrin, iron, and dermatophytes. I. Serum dematophyte inhibitory component definitively identified as unsaturated transferrin. *J. Lab. Clin. Med.*, 86, 204–212.

[120] Wakabayashi H, Takakura N, Yamauchi K, Teraguchi S, Uchida K, Yamaguchi H, Tamura Y. (2002). Effect of lactoferrin feeding on the host antifungal response in guinea-pigs infected or immunised with *Trichophyton mentagrophytes*. *J. Med. Microbiol.*, 51, 844–850.

[121] Rollins-Smith LA, Woodhams DC, Reinert LK, Vredenburg VT, Briggs CJ, Nielsen PF, Conlon JM. (2006). Antimicrobial peptide defenses of the mountain yellow-legged frog (Rana muscosa). *Develop. Comp. Immunol.*, 30, 831–842.

[122] Lopez-Garcia B, Lee, PH, Gallo RL. (2006). Expression and potential function of cathelicidin antimicrobial peptides in dermatophytosis and tinea versicolor. *J. Antimicrob. Chemother*, 57, 877–882.

[123] Davies RR, Zaini F. (1988). Drugs affecting *Trichophyton rubrum*-induced neutrophil chemotaxis *in vitro*. *Clin. Exp. Dermatol.*, 13, 228–231.

[124] Calderon RA, Hay RJ. (1987). Fungicidal activity of human neutrophils and monocytes on dermatophyte fungi, *Trichophyton quinckeanum* and *Trichophyton rubrum*. *Immunology*, 61, 289–296.

[125] Calderon RA, Shennan GI. (1987). Susceptibility of *Trichophyton quinckeanum* and *Trichophyton rubrum* to products of oxidative metabolism. *Immunology*, 61, 283–288.

[126] Graham JH, Barrosos-Tobila C. (1971). Dermatophytosis. In: *The Pathologic Anatomy of the Mycoses*, Baker, R. D., Ed., Springer, Berlin, pp. 211–235.

[127] Serrano-Gomez D, Leal JAC, Angel, L. (2005). DC-SIGN mediates the binding of *Aspergillus fumigatus* and keratinophylic fungi by human dendritic cells. *Immunobiology*, 210, 175–183.

[128] Calderon RA, Hay RJ. (1984). Cell-mediated immunity in experimental murine dermatophytosis. II. Adoptive transfer of immunity to dermatophyte infection by lymphoid cells from donors with acute or chronic infections. *Immunology*, 53, 465–472.

[129] Koga T. (2009). Fungal immunology in the skin; immune response to dermatophytes. *Nippon Ishinkin Gakkai Zasshi*, 50(3), 151-154.

[130] Nakamura Y, Kano R, Hasegawa A, Watanabe S. (2002). Interleukin-8 and tumor necrosis factor alpha production in human epidermal keratinocytes induced by *Trichophyton mentagrophytes*. *Clin. Diagn Lab. Immunol.,* 9(4), 935-937.

[131] Shiraki Y, Ishibashi Y, Hiruma M, Nishikawa A, Ikeda S. (2006). Cytokine secretion profiles of human keratinocytes during *Trichophyton tonsurans* and *Arthroderma benhamiae* infections. *J. Med. Microbiol.*, 55, 1175–1185.

[132] Raska M, Zemanova E, Kafkova L, Belakova J, Vudattu NK, Kopecek P, Weigl E. (2004). Isolation and characterization of an immunogenic fragment of heat shock protein 60 from *Trichophyton mentagrophytes*. *Mycoses*, 47, 482–490.

[133] Mignon B. (2005). New studies on the characterization of virulence factors in *Microsporum canis*. *Bull Mem. Acad. Royale Med. Belgique*, 160, 270–275.

[134] Calderon RA, Hay RJ, Shennan GI. (1987). Circulating antigens and antibodies in human and mouse dermatophytosis: use of monoclonal antibody reactive to phosphorylcholine-like epitopes. *J. Gen. Microbiol.*, 133, 2699–2705.

[135] Calderon RA. (1989). Immunoregulation of dermatophytosis. *Crit. Revs. Microbiol.*, 16, 339–368.

[136] Brasch J. Sterry W. (1992). Immunophenotypical characterization of inflammatory cellular infiltrates in tinea. *Act. Dermato. Venereol.*, 72, 345–347.

[137] Leibovici V, Evron R, Axelrod O, Westerman M, Shalit M, Barak V, Frankenburg S. (1995). Imbalance of immune responses in patients with chronic and widespread fungal skin infection.*Clin. Exp. Dermatol.*, 20, 390–394.

Chapter 4

IMMUNOMODULATION: TARGETING THE HOST

Manipulating the immune system by derivatives from specific pathogens (vaccines), pathogen-specific immune response components (Abs, phagocytes or T cells), or nonpathogen-specific immune response derivatives (cytokines and AMPs) is becoming an integral part in the prevention and treatment of viral and bacterial infections. They are also providing tools to better manage patients with cancer, allergy, autoimmunity and transplantation. In the case of fungal infections however, these preventive and therapeutic modalities are still in the basic research/development stage. There is mounting experimental evidence however to suggest that manipulating the immune response holds considerable promise to better manage and treat serious fungal infections. There is also evidence to suggest that host-targeting interventions can significantly enhance the outcome of conventional antifungal chemotherapy. The efficacy of vaccines, cytokines, adoptively transferred cells, and other such modalities in modulating immunity depends on their respective potential to direct and/or stimulate the immune response against fungal infections. In general terms therefore, their success in modulating immunity can only be limited by factors that block, dilute or undesirably amplify their activity. Hence, problems that classically associate with chemotherapy (narrow spectrum of activity, toxicity and resistance) can dramatically decrease. Nonetheless, blunted or overwhelmed immunity, pathogen-strain replacement, and the increased likelihood of inflammation can be potential spoilers. Both the advantages and disadvantages of antifungal immunomodulation will be discussed in subsequent sections of this chapter and in chapter 6.

VACCINES

The promise vaccines hold for enhancing our ability to control and manage fungal infections far exceeds that of any other preventive or therapeutic immunomodulatory approach. The sheer number of studies carried out towards this endeavor in comparison with that in other areas like adoptive cell transfer or cytokine therapy testifies to this effect. Although clinical trials of the coccidioidomycosis vaccine that were conducted in the 1980s by the Valley Fever Vaccine Study Group failed to yield significant differences in susceptibility to coccidioidomycosis between immunized and placebo subjects [1], these studies marked the true beginning of research work on fungal vaccines. Following these initial studies, the identification, development, and testing of various approaches and components related to fungal vaccine research has witnessed breathtaking advances. Unfortunately however, the vast majority of experimental fungal vaccines developed thus far have failed to fair any better than the coccidioidomycosis vaccine. Systematic review of approaches involved in the design, development and testing of experimental fungal vaccines is needed in order to define some of the obstacles hindering their progress. In attempting to address this issue, the following discussion will deal with classical and recombinant fungal vaccines as well as recent work on fungal vaccine adjuvants. Some of the forthcoming contributions of genomics and proteomics to fungal vaccine design and development will also be addressed.

Adjuvants

Maximizing the potential of success of a vaccine is dependent upon a number of factors. Chief among these is vaccine immunogenicity, lack of cross-reactivity with host antigens, and the use of compatible adjuvants. Use of adjuvants is essential to enhance the immune response to vaccines and induce long-term memory, especially when vaccines are prepared from whole killed organisms. Different classes of adjuvants that slowdown antigen degradation (depot adjuvants) like aluminum salts, deliver antigens to antigen presenting cells (APCs) (particulate adjuvants) like microparticles, iscoms, and liposomes, or stimulate immunity and promote cytokine production by activating APCs (immunostimulatory adjuvants) like lipopolysaccharides, microbial cytidylate-phosphate-guanylate DNA, and saponins are currently available. The efficacy of adjuvants is hard to predict; in other words, it can be said that achieving optimal vaccine/adjuvant combinations is a matter of trial and error. Developing new adjuvants or exploring different combinations from the depot/particulate pool and the immunostimulatory pool is complementary to the production of effective vaccines, fungal or otherwise. Overall, some of the adjuvants tested in conjunction with different fungal immunogenic moieties have proven useful. Subcutaneous immunization of *Candida albicans* membrane antigen (CMA) mixed with incomplete Freund's adjuvant induced resistance to infections caused by *C. albicans* and *A. fumigatus* in mice [2]. Immunoprotection of the *Candida*-derived rAls3p-N vaccine was enhanced when administered in combination with the depot adjuvant aluminum hydroxide [3]. Immunogenicity and efficacy of rAls3p-N plus aluminum hydroxide was greatly enhanced when diluted in phosphate-buffered saline as compared with that diluted in saline; this although the quantity of rAls3p-N bound to aluminum hydroxide was greater in the later diluent [4]. Use of immunostimulatory adjuvants has been associated with positive outcomes in experimental fungal vaccine studies [5-8]. For example, vaccination with the recombinant truncated form of the *A. fumigatus* antigen Aspf3 that lacks the IgE binding sites was protective against aspergillosis when mixed with TiterMax [9].

Enhanced immunostimulatory effects of bacterial DNA, which stems from the presence of CpG dinucleotide-rich sequences, has been utilized to develop a class of adjuvants known as CpG-oligodeoxynucleotides (CpG-ODNs). The therapeutic value of CpG-ODNs is dependent upon their ability to enhance the differentiation of Th1-mediated immune responsiveness. As CpG-ODNs induce Th1-type cytokines, some investigators [10] have speculated that they may suppress Th2-type responses, a beneficial outcome in allergy. Treatment of asthmatic patients with CpG-ODNs minimized injurious eosinophil-mediated inflammation [10]. CpG-ODNs have been used as adjuvants with experimental fungal vaccines. Enhanced capacity of the *A. fumigatus* Aspf16 antigen to protect against murine aspergillosis when mixed with unmethylated CpG-ODNs was attributed to the adjuvant's ability to engage Th1-mediated protective immunity [11-13]. Additionally, although treatment of mice with *C. neoformans* infection using fluconazole or unmethylated CpG-ODN improved survival, cleared the pathogen, and prevented dissemination, combined treatment using both agents significantly improved therapy outcome [14]. While the general consensus is that treatment with CpG-ODN confers protection and enhances resistance to a wide spectrum of fungal pathogens, some instances to the contrary have been reported. For example, treatment of normal mice with synthetic CpG-ODNs was shown to increase susceptibility to infection with resistant strains of *C. albicans* [15].

The enormous potential of DCs to recognize, process, and present fungal antigens and to orchestrate innate and adaptive immune responses against fungal infections has been employed in vaccine design and "adjuvanation" procedures [11, 12, 16-18]. As discussed previously, several effective immunostimulatory adjuvants that can engage adaptive CMI are available. However, the appeal of DC-based vaccine strategies derives from their ability to package immunogenicity into immunostimulatory rather than idle molecular entities. Fungal vaccine design dependent upon the use of DCs pulsed with whole fungi, fungal cell extracts or fungal RNA has been tried with some success [11]. Vaccination with *A. fumigatus* antigen extract-pulsed DCs mixed with CpG-ODN protected mice against subsequent *A. fumigatus* infections in a Th1-dependent manner [13]. Upregulation of several TLRs on DCs following pulsation with fungal RNA suggests that fungal RNA can activate DCs via nucleotide receptor signaling cascades [12]. Administration of *A. fumigatus* RNA-pulsed DCs induced Th1-derived IFN-γ-dependent protective responses against subsequent challenges with *A. fumigatus* [12]. Interestingly, the cytosine deaminase (CD) activity of DCs, which converts the antifungal 5-fluorocytosine (5-FC) into the potent anticancer compound 5-FU [19, 20], has been utilized to generate libraries of recombinant Ab fragments (mainly, single-chain variable fragments), display them on phage surfaces, and select phage Abs against target antigens for possible clinical use [21]. Use of pharmacologically-activated invariant natural killer T (iNKT) cells [22] or rapamycin-induced autophagy [23] were shown to positively modulate DCs and enhance antigen-specific B and T cell responses in the presence of immunogenic proteins.

Though not directly related to adjuvants, modifications involving the structure and/or composition of fungal antigens have been reported to significantly enhance vaccine immunogenicity *in vivo*. Immunization with the tetanus toxoid conjugate of glucuronoxylomannan (GXM) resulted in the production of protective Abs in animal models of cryptococcosis [24]. When diphtheria toxoid CRM197 is conjugated with the algal antigen laminarin (Lam), a *Laminaria digitata*–derived poorly immunogenic cell wall β-glucan, the resultant vaccine was protective against murine systemic and mucosal candidiasis [25]. Inclusion of the Lam antigen enabled a novel polysaccharide-protein conjugate vaccine to induce the production of Abs against β-glucan and to protect against experimental candidiasis and aspergillosis [26]. Thymosin α1 promoted dendritic cell (DC) activation and production of interleukin-12 (IL-12)p70 and interferon-gamma (IFN-γ) and enhanced the priming of Th1 responses against aspergillosis [27]. The ability of thymosin-α1 to activate *A. fumigatus*-pulsed DCs and in turn activate Th1-dependent fungal immunity, accelerate myeloid cell recovery, and protect highly susceptible mice should collectively qualify this toll like receptors 9 (TLR9) ligand as a strong candidate carrier that seems to coordinate the activation of innate and adaptive immunity [27, 28]. By using ovalbumin (OVA) expressed in bacterial and yeast vectors, it was demonstrated that fungal mannosylation enhances antigen immunogenicity in the context of $CD4^+$ T cell responses [29]. O-linked mannosylated yeast-derived OVA antigens were reported to be more potent than unmannosylated counterparts at inducing antigen-specific T cell proliferation [30]. Although neither O-linked nor N-linked mannosylated OVA antigens succeeded in stimulating DCs to produce TNF-α or IL-12, the ability of mannosylation to engage adaptive cell-mediated immunity (CMI) is nonetheless promising.

Classical Approaches to Fungal Vaccine Development

Notwithstanding the presence of considerable similarities between fungal and human cells (the presence of a nucleus surrounded by a nuclear membrane, 80S ribosomes, and Golgi apparatus as well as the use of similar mechanisms for DNA, RNA and protein synthesis among a whole host of similarities), the list of fungal cell antigens that are immunogenic in mammalian hosts is extensive [31, 32]. As the cell wall plays an important role in host-fungus interactions, several cell wall components are major inducers of fungal immunity, hence the interest in such components as potential candidates for vaccine development. For instance, vaccination with *C. albicans* β-mercaptoethanol (β-ME) extracts prolonged survival and decreased fungal burden in mice upon subsequent challenge with lethal doses of the pathogen [33]. Proteomic analysis has revealed the presence of complex polypeptide patterns with multiple immunogenic components associated with β-ME extracts that were used in the preparation of the vaccine. Immunization of rabbits with a glycolconjugate consisting of synthetic *C. albicans* β-1,2-mannan disaccharides clustered on a glucose core and conjugated with tetanus toxoid resulted in the generation of high titers of Abs reactive with the disaccharide cluster and the trisaccharide epitope [8]. Anti-sera from immunized rabbits cross-reacted with *C. albicans* β-mannan cell wall extracts. A glycolconjugate consisting of the *C. albicans*-expressed complement receptor 3-related protein (CR3-RP) has demonstrated significant immunogenic potential in rabbits [5]. *C. neoformans*, as an opportunistic fungus, causes life-threatening pneumonia and meningoencephalitis in immunocompromised patients. Immunization of BALB/c mice with the IFN-γ-inducing *C. neoformans* strain H99γ was shown to be protective against subsequent pulmonary challenges with lethal strains of *C. neoformans* [34]. Compared with heat-killed *C. neoformans*, which failed to induce protection against subsequent *C. neoformans* infections, immunization with the *C. neoformans* H99γ strain resulted in increased pulmonary granulomatous formation and leukocyte infiltration that resolved pulmonary inflammation and protected the lungs against severe allergic bronchopulmonary cryptococcosis. Mice deficient for IL-4 receptor, IL-12p40, IL-12p35, IFN-γ, or T cells failed to develop resistance to pulmonary challenge of the pathogen demonstrating the need for intact T cell immunity (Th1 in particular) for the vaccine to be protective. Th1-dependent protection of the vaccine was further demonstrated by the finding that production of Th1 proinflammatory cytokines and percentages and absolute numbers of $CD4^+$ T cells, $CD11c^+$ cells, and $Gr\text{-}1^+$ cells noticeably increased in immunized mice.

Sugar modifications can alter immunogenicity of fungal antigens [15, 16]. For example, it was reported that mannosylation of an immunoreactive cryptococcal mannoprotein was critical for optimal T cell responsiveness against *C. neoformans* [35]. Administration of a CR3-RP glycolconjugate triggered enhanced CMI by upregulating the expression of IL-2 receptor α-subunit (CD25) on B lymphocytes, induced isotype switching, and increased the $CD4^+/CD8^+$ ratio in hosts. Vaccination of BALB/c mice with the *C. albicans* ecm33 mutants (RML2U), mutants that express cell walls rich in protein in the outermost layer, was protective against subsequent lethal doses of the virulent *C. albicans* strain SC5314 [6]. The *Candida* rAls3p-N vaccine, a variant of the rAls1p-N vaccine, was shown to be effective when combined with aluminum hydroxide adjuvant [3]. Although immunoprotection conferred by rAls3p-N vaccine was comparable to that induced by rAls1p-N against disseminated candidiasis, the new variant vaccine was superior to rAls1p-N in protecting against oropharyngeal and vaginal candidiasis [36]. While intraperitoneally-administered rAls1p-N modestly improved survival during disseminated candidiasis in mice, increased efficacy was achieved by using the subcutaneous route. In a mouse model of brain cryptococcosis, intracerebral administration of doubly-treated heat-inactivated *C. neoformans* cells enhanced survival after subsequent local challenge with lethal doses of *C. neoformans*. Survival was associated with local inflammation, reduced fungal growth within the brain and development of delayed-type hypersensitivity (DTH) [37].

Immunization of BALB/c mice with radio-attenuated *Paracoccidioides brasiliensis* cells promoted lasting protection against virulent forms of the pathogen as >99% decrease in colony forming unit (CFU) recovery was evident three months post challenge [38]. The protective effects of this experimental vaccine were associated with Th1-mediated responses; namely increased levels of IgG2a and IFN-γ production. Treatment of dexamethasone-anergized *P. brasiliensis*-infected BALB/c mice with a 15mer peptide from the major diagnostic antigen gp43 (P10) in combination with chemotherapy reduced lung fungal burden and prevented fungal dissemination to liver and spleen [39]. Previously, it has been shown that vaccination with P13, a decapeptide mimotope of the cryptococcal capsular polysaccharide GXM protects against subsequent lethal *C. neoformans* challenges [40, 41]. In chronically infected mice, vaccination with P13 prolonged survival and upregulated the expression of IFN-γ, IL-6 and IL-10 in a manner dependent on mouse strain (BALB/c vs C57BL/6), carrier protein type (tetanus toxoid vs diphtheria toxoid) and route of infection (intraperitoneal vs intravenous) [42]. Follow-up studies on the efficacy of the gp43 vaccine have demonstrated that while immunization of BALB/c mice with gp43 alone resulted in the generation of strong gp43-specific IgG1 responses coupled with the secretion of IL-4 and IL-10. Intranasal administration of the P10 peptide fused to a recombinant *Salmonella enterica*-derived FliC flagellin, a TLR5-binding agonist, elicited robust Th1 type immune responses [43]. In a related recent study [44] however, mAbs generated against a heptasaccharide representing the major structural motif of GMX (M2) that is present in common clinical isolates of *C. neoformans* failed to elicit protective Ab responses. Based on these findings it was concluded that the M2 motif of *C. neoformans* GXM moiety is not suitable for vaccination purposes. A 25KD cryptococcal deacetylase (d25) was able to induce cell proliferation and secretion of IL-2 and IFN-γ, but not IL-4, in spleen cells isolated from mice immunized with the d25 or infected with *C. neoformans* [45]. Secretion of IFN-γ, but not IL-2, was essential for anti-cryptococcosis activity of d25 in mice [45].

Synthetic chemistry has been a considerable source of chemically-defined immunogenes that can be used to design experimental fungal vaccines. A novel, immunologically neutral, linker methodology to prepare highly defined vaccine conjugates has been recently described [46]. This methodology relies on combining complex saccharide antigens with specific Th cell epitopes. Using this method, two glycoconjugates prepared from synthetic (1→2)-β-mannan trisaccharide with inter residue-S-linked mannopyranose residues and coupled to tetanus toxoid elicited the synthesis of Abs that recognize O-linked trisaccharide epitopes in native cell wall antigens of *C. albicans* [7]. Using this saccharide-peptide linker chemistry, T cell peptides from *C. albicans* wall proteins were synthesized and conjugated to the cell wall beta-mannan trisaccharide (beta-(Man)(3). Out of six glycopeptide conjugates, three (beta-(Man)(3)-Fba, -Met6, and -Hwp1) were able to increase survival and reduce kidney fungal burden in mice with candidiasis [47]. The other three conjugates either moderately protected against (-Eno1 and -Gap1) or slightly enhanced disease (-Pgk1).

Cross-Kingdom Vaccines

Using antigenic components derived from one strain or species to vaccinate against a related strain or species is relatively common in preparing viral and bacterial vaccines. Vaccination across higher orders of classification is not that uncommon either. For example, CD-1 mice receiving weekly injections of heat-killed *S. cerevisiae* (HKY) via the subcutaneous or oral routs prior to the initiation of coccidioidomycosis experienced prolonged survival and reduced fungal burden [48]. In contrast, vaccination across different life kingdoms has been uncommon until recently [49]. The algal beta-glucan (laminarin) vaccine when conjugated with an appropriate protein component (diphtheria toxoid CRM197) was protective against a wide array of fungal infections through the induction of Abs that inhibit fungal growth [50]. Based on the relative success of laminarin and other preparations in experimental animal models it has been argued that, with some fine-tuning, it may become possible to use preparations like laminarin to vaccinate against classes of fungal pathogens expressing the beta-glucan moiety [49]. Vaccination with the recombinant N terminus of the *Candida* adhesin Als3p (rAls3p-N) was protective against lethal candidemia [3, 51, 52] and *S. aureus* infections especially when combined with aluminum hydroxide [53]. The cross-kingdom protective potential of Als3p was attributed to shared similarities with the *S. aureus*-derived clumping factor. In the reverse direction however, the protective potential of *S. aureus* clumping factor against candidiasis is yet to be fully explored. Several putative major histocompatibility molecule (MHC)-II-binding proteins deduced from *E. coli* by proteomic and/or bioinformatic means were also reported to be protective against *Coccidiodes posadasii* infections in mice [54]. Although initial hype regarding rAg2/Pra (a bacterially-expressed recombinant proline-rich protein) as a potential *Candida* vaccine has subsided due to contradictory data, subsequent promising findings have been reported [55]. In that, subcutaneous vaccination of C57BL/6 or BALB/c mice with rAg2/Pra plus an adjuvant followed by intraperitoneal challenge with *C. posadasii* significantly reduced fungal burden. When mixed with an adjuvant, a combined vaccine consisting of rAg2/Pra and a *C. posadasii*-derived molecular homologue (Prp2) sharing 69% sequence identity with rAg2/Pra was able to induce significant T cell-mediated protection against intranasal challenge with *C. posadasii*. This protective effect was attributed to the capacity of the combined vaccine to stimulate a heterogeneous T-cell repertoire as compared with the relatively homogeneous response generated by rAg2/Pra vaccine alone [55].

Recombinant Vaccines

Work on recombinant fungal vaccines, which has been going on for some time now, is extensive in terms of approaches, target pathogens and outcomes. However, the overall success of this approach in delivering effective fungal vaccines still falls way short of the fan-fair with which it has started. That is not to say that the promise is totally lost. In fact, the following discussion will try to make this very point by citing random examples, albeit recent, from across the board. Vaccination with a recombinant strain of *Blastomyces dermatiditis* lacking the WI-1 adhesin gene was reported to be protective against pathogenic strains of the fungus through Th1-mediated responses [56]. Significant humoral immune responses were noted following immunization with HSP90 constituents, recombinant HSP90 protein preparations or HSP90-encoding DNA vaccines administered via the intradermal, intranasal, or intravenous routes [57]. Priming by an intradermal injection of rHSP90 followed by intranasal or intradermal boosting with the same form significantly increased serum and vaginal fluid concentration of *Candida* HSP90-specific IgG and IgA Abs and enhanced HSP90-specific splenocyte responses *in vitro*. Immunization of C57BL/6J mice with a hybrid phage consisting of *C. albicans* HSP90 DEPAGE specific epitope (SE-CA-HSP90) expressed on a filamentous phage surface and fused to a major phage coat protein (pVIII) was able to reduce kidney fungal burden, induce anti-SE-CA-HSP90 Ab responses, enhance DTH responses, enhance NK cell activity, and augment ConA-induced splenocyte proliferation [58]. Immunization with a *C. albicans* HSP90 protein-expressing DNA vaccine cloned into the vaccination vector pVAX1 was able to protect against systemic candidiasis in BALB/c mice by eliciting the production of protective anti-*Candida*-HSP90 IgG Abs [59]. A recombinant HSP90-related protein 60 (rHSP60) was able to reduce fungal burden and induce synthesis of IFN-γ and IL-12 in mice with *P. brasiliensis* [60]. Immunization with the *H. capsulatum* cell surface protein HSP60, which represents a key target of cell-mediated immunity during histoplasmosis, was also shown to be protective [61].

The protective potential of a genetically engineered *C. albicans* tet-NRG1 strain-derived antigen tested as an experimental live, attenuated vaccine against disseminated candidiasis was shown to be dependent upon T cell immunity both in immunocompetent and immunodeficient mice [62]. Immunization with a recombinant antigen of *A. fumigatus* (rAspf3) was protective against invasive aspergillosis [63]. Three truncated versions of rAspf3, spanning amino acid residues 15-168, 1-142 and 15-142 (all lacking sequences required for IgE binding) were also protective. Interestingly, vaccination with rAspf3 (1–142) or rAspf3 (15–168) drastically diminished the production of antigen-specific Abs compared with the full-length rAspf3 (1–168) or the double-truncate rAspf3 (15–142). These findings suggest that it is possible to design vaccines that target cellular immunity and activate T cells capable of enhancing the function of macrophages or other cellular elements involved in fungal pathogen clearance. In search for additional *Aspergillus* immunogenic antigens, a λ-phage cDNA expression library prepared from *A. fumigatus* mRNA was used to screen for *A. fumigatus* antigens reactive with anti-sera from rabbits infected with conidiospores of *A. fumigatus*. Abs against several antigens including the glycosylhydrolase Asp-f-16, enolase, and HSP90 were produced by recipient rabbits [64]. A cDNA library constructed from *A. fumigatus* mycelia using the λ-ZAP expression vector and tested against sera from patients with allergic bronchopulmonary aspergillosis (ABPA) revealed the presence of a novel gene encoding the 43KD *A. fumigatus* allergen Aspf16. Aspf16 was able to react with IgE from ABPA patients but not with sera from patients with allergic asthma, asymptomatic *Aspergillus* skin test-positive asthmatics or normal controls [65]. The Aspf16 allergen was also able to induce significant proliferation in peripheral blood mononuclear (PBM) cells isolated from patients with ABPA. The deduced amino acid sequence of Aspf16 shares extensive sequence homology with a 31KD antigen known as Aspf9 [65-67]. Vaccination with a recombinant form of Aspf3 or with a truncated form of Aspf3 lacking the IgE binding sites was protective against aspergillosis [12]. The protective potential of truncated Aspf3 was dependent upon the presence of the adjuvant TiterMax.

Vaccination with a recombinant N-terminal domain of A1s1p (rA1s1p-N) was protective against disseminated candidiasis in BALB/c and other outbred mouse strains [68]. As Aspf3 and related molecules and truncates can stimulate adaptive CMI and as these molecular entities exist in other *Aspergillus* species and other molds (*Coccidioides posadasii* and *Penicillium citrinum*), and yeasts (*C. albicans*, *C. boidinii* and *S. cerevisiae*), it is worth testing the capacity of Aspf3 and related structures and homologues to act as pan-fungal (or cross-genera) vaccines.

A genetically-engineered, live, attenuated vaccine constructed by disrupting two chitinase genes (CTS2 and CTS3) of *C. posadasii* or *C. immitis* was recently shown to be protective against coccidioidomycosis in BALB/c and C57BL/6 mice [69]. Vaccinated animals mounted immune responses involving the production of Th1 and Th2 type cytokines that collectively helped to establish well-formed granulomas, diminish infection-associated inflammation and reduce lung fungal burden. As mentioned previously, Pcp is a prevalent opportunistic infection among AIDS patients worldwide. Alveolar macrophages recognize Pc through a Pc β-glucan C-type lectin receptor known as dectin-1. Treatment of SCID mice with Pcp using a fusion protein consisting of the extracellular domain of dectin-1 plus murine IgG1 Fc fragment reduced lung fungal burden and tissue damage [70]. The protective effect of dectine-1-Fc was related to its ability to enhance macrophage recognition of β-glucan and its capacity to opsonize Pc cells for killing by alveolar macrophages. DCs and macrophages from dectin-1-deficient mice failed to produce cytokines in response to stimulation by β-glucan *in vitro* [70].

The *-Omics* Promise

The availability of complete genome sequences of more than 90 different fungal species including *C. albicans*, *A. fumigatus*, and *S. cerevisiae* among others is making it possible to revise previously published gene sequences of fungal proteins currently available at different data bases such as Genebank and IUIS. A study that has compared old published sequences of many proteins with updated genome sequences concluded that there could be a core set of allergen-like proteins in each fungal species [71]. The study identified a number of inconsistencies in the approved allergen list available at Genebank and IUIS data bases. It concluded that Aspf 56KD (Aspf15) and (Aspf16) ought to be replaced by the larger protein motif (Aspf17). Additionally, the study suggested that Aspf12 ought to be classified as HSP90, Mala s 10 as hsp88 and (Alt a 3, Cla h 4 and Pen c 19) as HSP70. Immunoproteomic and bioinformatic approaches to deduce pathogen-derived proteins capable of binding with MHC molecules (MHC-II in particular) and able to stimulate Th cell-mediated protective immunity has resulted in the discovery of *Escherichia coli*–derived putative proteins protective against Coccidiomycosis in C57BL/6 mice [54]; another potential cross-kingdom vaccine. Twenty nine *C. albicans*–derived immunoreactive proteins that specifically react with Abs from vaccinated mouse sera were identified using immunoproteomic approaches [6]. Six of these proteins (Gnd1p, Cit1p, Rpl10Ep, Yst1p, Cys4p, Efb1p) were described as immunogenic. Proteins that were exclusively identified in the mutant surfome (Met6p, Eft2p, Tkl1p, Rpl10Ep, Atp1p, Atp2p) were also immunogenic [6]. In summary, while still in its infancy with regard to fungal pathogens, diseases and immunotherapetics, the *–omics* revolution may prove valuable in identifying infinite numbers of fungal antigens and peptides as potential immunotherapeutic candidates. Devising high contrast *in silico* and *in vitro* screening strategies to drastically minimize the number of molecules worthy of further evaluation is essential should the voluminous data generated by fungal genomic and proteomic research not become a major distraction.

CELL TRANSFER THERAPY

Cells of innate and adaptive immunity are pivotal in mediating protection against fungal infections. Using cellular components to prime, modulate, and enhance immunity against fungi is one of the approaches being developed and tested to treat fungal infections. Work on this front has focused on using mixed or purified pools of cells (DCs, NK cells, $CD4^+$ T cells and $CD8^+$ T cells) either isolated from infected animals or manipulated *in vitro* prior to their application as non-adaptive or adaptive immunotherapeutic modulators. Work on the transfer of DCs has already been described in the previous section; therefore, the discussion below will mainly deal with experimental work pertinent to mixture cell populations, phagocytes, NK cells, and T lymphocytes.

It has been reported that pharmacologically-activated iNKT cells can positively modulate DCs and enhance antigen-specific B and T cell responses in the presence of antigenic proteins [29]. Human lymphocytes cultured with IL-2 were shown to conjugate with and directly inhibit the growth of various strains of *C. neoformans* [72]. Highly purified populations of human lymphocytes cultured with encapsulated *C. neoformans* exhibited strong fungistatic activity involving NK, $CD4^+$, $CD8^+$, and $CD16/56^+$ T cells [73]. Besides the capacity of Aspf16 antigen to induce humoral and allergic responses against *Aspergillus* [63-65], it can induce effector T cell responses. In that, *Aspergillus*-specific cytotoxic T lymphocytes (CTLs) were generated from PBM cell cultures stimulated by DCs pulsed with the complete pool of pentadecapeptides (PPCs) spanning the coding region of Aspf16 or stimulted by APCs consisting of Epstein-Barr virus (EBV)-transformed B lymphoblastoid cells (BLCL) [24]. PPC-DC-only-primed cell lines induced effector cell phenotype and peptide specificity at levels comparable to those of DC/BLCL primed cell lines. However, the later approach was more efficient in generating Aspf16-specific IFN-γ-producing cells at higher frequency. Administration of DCs pulsed with the overlapping pentadecapeptides spanning the entire 427-aa coding region of Aspf16 induced strong proliferative responses [74]. A $CD4^+$ IFN-γ producing cell line isolated from immunized donors was cytotoxic to autologous pool-pulsed and *Aspergillus* culture extract-pulsed targets. Furthermore, two lines isolated from HLA-$B*3501^+$ donors following challenge with DCs pulsed with the overlapping pentadecapeptides were strongly cytotoxic to autologous target cells pulsed with either Aspf16-peptide pool or *Aspergillus* culture extracts [75]. Culture supernatants from these cell lines exhibited considerable killing activity against *Aspergillus* conidia. Moreover, cells from these cultures exhibited direct cytotoxic activity against *Aspergillus* hyphae. MHC I (HLA-B*3501)-restricted $CD8^+$ T cells were exclusively responsible for the cytotoxic activity and IFN-γ production [75]. While use of B cells or serum from animals immunized with *Candida*-derived rAls3p-N antigen failed to transfer protection to naive animals as Ab titers were lower than baseline values (> or = 1:6400), adoptive transfer of $CD3^+$, $CD4^+$ or $CD8^+$ T cells from immunized mice was protective against candidiasis in naïve mice [3]. Based on the assumption that Th cells are of significance in inducing anti-aspergillosis immunity, especially in hematopoietic stem cell transplant (HSCT) patients, a method of large-scale generation of anti-aspergillosis T cells has been recently described [76, 77]. In this study, about 10^9 white blood cells were stimulated with *Aspergillus* antigens; IFN-γ producing cells were selected and expanded. Within two weeks, a median number of $2x10^7$ $CD3^+CD4^+$ cells exhibiting an activated memory Th phenotype were obtained. Upon re-stimulation, there was significant *in vitro* Th1 differentiation as evidenced by the presence of significant numbers of viable T cells secreting IFN-γ, but no IL-4 or IL-10.

This technique may be useful in prospective trials for large-scale adoptive transfer of fungal antigen-primed T cells.

Adoptive transfer of $CD4^+$ splenocytes from mice sensitized with *A. fumigatus* into naïve mice was shown to prolong survival following intravenous challenge with viable *A. fumigatus* conidia [66]. Following stimulation with cell wall or membrane components of *B. dermatitidis*, $CD4^+$ T cells expressing $V\alpha2^+J\alpha49^+$ and $V\beta^+J\beta1^+$ TCR antigens but not those expressing $V\beta8.1^+$ or $V\beta8.2^+$ were able to adoptively transfer protective immunity and produce high levels of IFN-γ. This finding suggests that the generation of protective T cell clones against immunodominant antigens of *B. dermatitidis* is greatly influenced by the TCRα and TCRβ combinations that favor the production of Th1 cytokine responses [78]. Along these lines, we have reported a pattern of time-dependent overexpansion of specific TCRVβ clones in a mouse model of estrogen-dependent vaginal candidiasis (EDVC) [79]. In that, T cell clones expressing TCRVβs 1, 6, 10 and 15 predominated during the intermediate phase (week 2) post *C. albicans* infection while those expressing TCRVβs 1, 4, 6, 8.3, 10, 13, 14 and 18 dominated the vaginal T cell pool at week 3 post infection. Moderately reduced tissue (lungs, spleen and liver) fungal burden was reported in nude C57BL/10 mice and 5Gy-irradiated heterozygous nude (nu/C57BL/6) mice intranasally challenged with *H. capsulatum* upon receiving an intravenous inoculation of resting 2.3H3 cells (a $CD4^+$ T cell clone) [80]. The effect was species-specific as mice challenged with *C. immitis* failed to clear the infection. These findings suggest that nude mice are permissive for the expression of adoptively-transferred anti-*H. capsulatum* T cell-mediated immunity. These and numerous similar findings call for further exploration of the potential of adoptively-transferred antigen-specific Th cells to modulate and restore protective immunity, especially in the immunocompromised.

$CD8^+$ T cell involvement in protection against infection is generally dependent upon help from Th cells. However, there is evidence to suggest that $CD8^+$ T cells play a significant role in protection against fungal infections in the absence of Th cell help. For instance, although CD4 deficiency impairs $CD8^+$ T cell activation and function in viral and bacterial infections [81, 82], generation of *C. neoformans*-specific effector $CD8^+$ T cells capable of producing protective levels of IFN-γ was reported to occur in CD4-deficient mice with pulmonary cryptococcosis [83]. The functionality of $CD8^+$-derived IFN-γ was demonstrated by the finding that neutralization of IFN-γ in $CD4^-$ $CD8^+$ mice increased macrophage susceptibility to infection by *C. neoformans*. Furthermore, IFN-γ, as the signature protective cytokine in the majority of fungal infections, seems to derive not only from Th1 cells but also from cells of phenotypes other than $CD4^+$ altogether. For example, depletion of $CD4^+$ T cells in mice treated with anti-CD40/IL-2 did not significantly diminish the concentration of serum IFN-γ [84]. Hence, the potential of $CD8^+$ cells to manipulate immunity against fungal infections is worth considering.

In addition to cell transfer work on lymphocyte, several studies have indicated that transfusion of donor granulocytes (neutrophils) is effective in alleviating the side effects of neutropenia and in enhancing the repopulation of granulocyte cell subsets [85-91]. Limitations on the potential benefits of G-CSF-mobilized granulocyte transfusion (GTX) treatment in neutropenic cancer patients derive from the fact that this form of treatment is often delayed for concerns of pulmonary reactions. However, these concerns have been recently challenged. In that, treatment of three children suffering from hematological malignancies and proven fungal infections (cerebral mold infection, disseminated candidiasis or nasopharyngeal mucormycosis) with combination antifungal therapy plus GTX during subsequent neutropenia effectively resolved the infections thus permitting anticancer therapy completion without delay [85]. A similar approach was successfully used to treat thirty two cancer patients with fungal infections [86]. A prospective phase II clinical trial was conducted to test the safety and efficacy of early-onset therapy using G-CSF-elicited cross-matched GTX therapy given at two doses consisting each of $8x10^8$ granulocytes/Kg body weight in neutropenic children with severe infections [87]. Results from the study suggest that early-onset GTX therapy is well-tolerated, does not result in notable pulmonary reactions, and is effective (>92% response rate) in clearing associated infections. Short-term activation ($\leq$3 days) and low dose irradiation of the human myeloid cell line (HL-60) was shown to generate viable, poorly replicative cells with candidacidal activity suitable for use as a novel GTX therapy [88]. Infusion of HL-60 cells treated in this manner significantly improved survival of neutropenic mice with candidemia. Reconstitution of neutrophil count and function by infusing G-CSF-activated GTX was reported to be effective at clearing *Zygomycete* infections [89]. In a recent clinical study, the efficacy and tolerability of 778 granulocyte transfusion procedures in 70 treatment episodes of neutropenic patients (49 children and 10 young adults) suffering from bacterial and/or fungal infections were assessed [91]. The study concluded that, with sufficient cell doses and rapid availability, granulocyte transfusion procedures can be helpful in treating neutroppenic patients with opportunistic infections. The study has also concluded that such procedures are safe given that adverse reactions like fever, chills, and mild pulmonary complications were rare. A phase III clinical trial sponsored by the National Institutes of Health (Heart, Lung, and Blood Institute) to evaluate the safety and efficacy of GTX in treating patients with bacterial and fungal infections during neutropenia is currently underway (*www.clinicaltrials.gov, Identifier: NCT00627393*).

It is clear from the preceding discussion that the search for immunotherapeutics in this area has focused on localized and systemic components of secondary, but not primary, lymphoid organs. It is well established that primary lymphoid organs are subject to significant infection-related structural and functional alterations. For instance, different types of pathogens infect the thymus and cause changes in the development and behavior of thymus-derived T cells [reviewed in 92]. During viral [93-95], bacterial [96, 97], fungal [98, 99], and protozoal [100, 101] infections, the thymus experiences atrophy, depletion of immature $CD4^{+}CD8^{+}$ cells, diminished thymocyte proliferation, epithelial network densification, and increased extracellular matrix deposition. Potential consequences of this process involve the induction of central tolerance to pathogen-derived antigens [92, 102] and the consequent generation of perturbed T cell repertoires containing autoreactive T cells and/or lacking T cell specificities needed to recognize and handle specific pathogens. In such cases, adoptive transfer of pathogen-specific T cells is an option; with that however comes potential cross-reactivity and immune responsiveness. The introduction of genetically-engineered syngeneic T cells expressing TCR specificities capable of handling a specific pathogen may be a more guided approach. However, this requires the identification of pathogen specific TCRαβ and/or TCRγδ T cell repertoires, a task which has already started [78, 79] but yet to be fully explored.

Cytokine Therapy

Based on current understanding of T cell immunity against fungal infections, it is postulated [31] that the relative significance of different T cell subsets in protection against fungal infections is dependent more on the cytokine profile they produce and less on their static phenotypic profile, vis-à-vis CD4 vs CD8 or, for that matter, lymphocytes vs phagocytes. Consequently, the use of proinflammatory, anti-inflammatory, regulatory, or suppressor cytokines to modulate the immune response during fungal infections seems the more logical. The ease with which optimal doses of cytokine therapy can be determined and effectively administered and the relative accessibility in managing potential adverse consequences adds to the fundamental appeal of cytokines as effective yet relatively benign agents with antifungal potential. Cytokine therapy may however be hampered by the need to maintain a delicate balance between inflammatory and anti-inflammatory cytokines so as to effectively fight infections without causing injurious inflammation [13, 103-106]. Cytokines are signaling molecules that specifically induce the proliferation, differentiation, activation, or suppression of target cells. In turn, cytokines specifically modulate host immunity in varied ways depending on the specific cytokine(s) involved, the subset of target cells expressing the respective receptor(s), the kinetics of interaction between the cytokine and its receptor, and the subsequent signaling cascade(s) generated by the interaction. Although the efficacy of antifungal cytokine therapy varies depending on the level and nature of immunosuppression or immunodeficiency and the antifungal agent being used to treat the infection, the benefits of cytokine therapy on the general outcome of managing mycotic infections is tangible. The pharmaceutical industry, having realized this, is hot on the trail for cytokine-based therapies against invasive fungal infections. For example, Leukine® (sargramostim; Bayer HealthCare Pharmaceuticals) is a GM-CSF preparation that is currently undergoing expanded evaluation (phase III clinical trial) as an antimycotic agent.

Administration of IFN-γ, IL-12 or anti-IL-4 can enhance Th1-dependent immunity against opportunistic fungal infections [107]. In an experimental model of cytokine gene therapy [108], it was demonstrated that J774 macrophages transfected with a single-chain cDNA encoding the p40 and p35 subunits of IL-12 construct can secrete biologically active IL-12 *in vitro*. Treatment of *C. immitis*–infected BALB/c mice (highly susceptible to coccidioidomycosis) with IL-12-transduced J774 cells inhibited *C. immitis* growth. The protective effects of IL-12-transduced J774 cells were correlated with a significant increase in IFN-γ synthesis in the lungs and blood of infected/treated mice. The immunotherapeutic role of IL-12 against *P. carinii* infection was demonstrated in IL-12 (p35)-deficient mice or mice depleted of $CD4^+$ cells [109]. Pathogen challenge followed by treatment with local IL-12 instillation or IL-12 gene therapy resulted in a rapid release of IL-12 into lung tissues and accelerated pathogen clearance from the lungs in normal mice. IL-12-deficient mice and mice depleted of $CD4^+$ cells showed delayed clearance of infection. Treatment of deficient or depleted mice with intranasal recombinant IL-12 accelerated clearance of the *P. carinii* infection. This response was associated with increased recruitment of inflammatory cells into lavage fluid and increased release of TNF-α, IL-12 and IFN-γ. Treatment with anti-CD40 in combination with IL-12 prolonged survival and protected mice against systemic cryptococcosis [84]. Protection in this model was correlated with decreased kidney and brain fungal burden and increased IFN-γ and TNF-α production. A similar treatment approach failed to protect IFN-γ knockout mice ($IFN\text{-}\gamma^{-/-}$) against *C. neoformans* infections suggesting that protection against cryptococcosis is IFN-γ-dependent. In a subsequent study, it was demonstrated that similar treatment regimens augmented host immunity against *C. neoformans* brain infections [110]. Protection in this case was correlated with upregulated MHC-II expression on brain $CD45^{low}CD11b^{+}$ cells and overall activation of microglial cells. Once again, IFN-γ was shown to be critical for microglial cell activation and anticryptococcal activity following treatment with anti-CD40/IL-2 combination albeit independent of $CD4^{+}$ T cell involvement [110].

Besides the well established protective roles of IFN-γ and IL-12 against fungal infections, some studies have suggested that IL-17 plays a positive role in regulating innate and adaptive immune responses against some forms of mycosis [reviewed in 111 and references therein]. IL-17, as a proinflammatory cytokine, was shown to induce the synthesis of downstream cytokines such as GM-CSF and CXCL8/IL-8 by localized differentiated neutrophils. Additionally, IL-17 can induce the synthesis of β-defensins and other AMPs. $CD4^{-}8^{-}TCR\alpha\beta^{+}$ or $TCR\gamma\delta^{+}$ T cells (mainly residents of the epithelium of the skin, GI and reproductive tracts) produce significant quantities of IL-17 [112, 113]. It has been reported that the duration of neutropenia was shortened following the administration of recombinant G-CSF and GM-CSF [114, 115]. Additionally, the phagocytic and killing activities of neutrophils, monocytes and macrophages were enhanced following the administration of recombinant G-CSF, M-CSF and GM-CSF [114, 115].

Administration of cytokines has proven beneficial when used in combination with chemotherapy. For example, cytokine adjunctive therapy of cancer patients with corticosteroid-induced neutropenia reduced the duration of neutropenia and enhanced granulcocyte antifungal activity, which minimized the risk of invasive fungal infections and permitted aggressive cytotoxic therapy [116]. Intranasal administration of GM-CSF into immunosuppressed mice suffering from pulmonary aspergillosis significantly reduced lung fungal burden suggesting that lung-targeted immunotherapy may complement antifungal chemotherapy and improve treatment outcome [117]. In mice with 5-FC-induced neutropenia, treatment with G-CSF augmented the antifungal activity of 5-FC. GM-CSF significantly enhanced polymorphonuclear cells (PMNs) fungicidal activity and enhanced the collaboration between PMNs and voriconazole or fluoconazole to kill *C.*

albicans [118]. However, the synergistic effect of GM-CSF was more evident in the case of voriconazole given that it is a more potent (>10-fold) anti-*Candida* azole than fluoconazole. G-CSF was shown to reverse neutrophil dysfunction against *Aspergillus* hyphae in HIV-infected non-neutropenic patients [119]. In cancer patients with therapy-refractory neutropenia, the response to antifungal therapy or even donor-derived GTX therapy is often suboptimal. Immune enhancement using recombinant IFN-1β in neutropenic cancer patients on G-CSF-stimulated GTX therapy successfully cleared or stabilized associated opportunistic fungal infections with minor side effects [90].

In this context, it is worth noting that conventional antifungals like polyenes (AMB and NY) and azoles (voriconazole and ketokonazole) can induce proinflammatory cytokine production and alter gene expression in different tissues. For example, upon recognition of AMB by TLR-2, several proinflammatory cytokines are released by TLR^{+} phagocytes [120, 121]. Furthermore, recognition and binding of NY by TLR-1- or TLR-2 has been reported to induce phagocytes to release several proinflammatory cytokines (IL-1β, IL-8 and TNF-α) [122]. As discussed previously, following recognition and binding of *A. fumigatus*-, *C. albicans*-, or *C. neoformans*-derived pathogen-associated molecular patterns (PAMPs) by TLRs 2, 4, 9 or CD14 on professional phagocytes an inflammatory response that induces Th1-mediated protective immunity ensues [13]. The capacity of polyenes to mimic fungal antigens and engage innate immunity in a TLR-dependent manner should provide new means to further explore the utility of cytokine therapy against fungal infections. While stimulation of THP-1 human MNs by *A. fumigatus* hyphal fragments alone caused significant upregulation in the activity of few cytokine genes (e.g. CCL4), co-stimulation with the fungal fragment and voriconazole resulted in upregulation of a larger number of cytokine/chemokine genes (CCLs 3, 4, 5, 7, 11 and 15 as well as CXCL6). This finding indicates that voriconazole enhances the capacity of fungal antigens to upregulate the expression of a wider and presumably more protective profile of cytokine genes [123]. Using a toxicogenomic microarray platform comprised of cDNA probes generated from mouse livers exposed to different hepatotoxicants, it was shown that out of 2364 genes assessed, ketoconazole at hepatotoxic doses upregulated nine genes encoding enzymes involved in phase I metabolism and one phase II enzyme (glutathione S-transferase) [124].

Immunosuppressants that target proinflammatory cytokines interfere with normal inflammatory and immune responses leading to increased incidence of opportunistic infections. Tissue availability and concentration permitting, some cytokine inhibitors bind target cytokines with high enough affinity to block binding with their respective receptors. Treatment with the TNF-α antagonists infliximab, adalimumab and the receptor fusion protein etanercept (FDA-approved drugs for the treatment of Crohn's disease, rheumatoid arthritis, psoriasis and other inflammatory diseases) has been associated with increased risk of bacterial and fungal infections [125-127]. The potential of certain cytokines to induce immunosuppression and other adverse effects has also been reported with regard to fungal infections. For example, administration of recombinant human G-CSF prior to infection with *A. fumigatus* in outbred ICR mice pretreated with hydrocortisone enhanced the action of the SCH56592 azole derivative [128]. However, it failed to be protective as treated mice developed large lung abscesses with significant PMN cell infiltration and high fungal burden. By removing G-CSF from the treatment regimen, reduced lung fungal burden and longer survival rates were observed.

Immunostimulatory Antibodies and Antifungal Peptides

As will be discussed in the next section, Ab- and AMP-based therapies, for the most part, target and neutralize and/or kill pathogens. However, there are cases where such molecules, whether generated as part of the immune response or administered as immunotherapeutics, can modulate host immunity. Development and use of molecules that can modulate and enhance protective immunity is desirable especially when Th differentiation does not move along the protective Th1 pathway, excessive inflammation, or selective immunodeficiency among other scenarios. In such cases, these and other molecules like cytokine inhibitors [125, 126], ligand-receptor inhibitors [84], and signaling molecules can be considered as constituents of the general class of host-targeting immunomodulatory agents [84, 125, 126, 129].

A protective natural mAb (3B4) that recognizes a surface antigen on *C. albicans* germ tubes was generated using B cells from *C. albicans*–infected mice [130]. Besides its pathogen-targeting role of suppressing germ tube formation, 3B4 was able to modulate phagocytosis and bind with the self-antigen keratin, which was shown to enhance the selection of B cells into the B1 B cell compartment, the site of antifungal Ab synthesis. An IgG1 mAb generated against a 70KD glycoprotein antigen secreted by the thermally dimorphic fungus *Sporothrix schenckii* significantly reduced CFU counts in an IFN-γ-dependent manner when injected before, during or after *S. schenckii* infection in immunocompetent or T cell-deficient mice [131]. The protective potential of anti-CD40 treatment against systemic *C. neoformans* infections has been correlated with increased IFN-γ and TNF-α production and upregulated expression of MHC-II on brain microglial cells [84].

With regard to AMPs, it is well established that ribotoxin-derived peptides, cathelicidins and other cationic peptides can modulate cytokine production, alter host gene expression profiles and minimize proinflammatory responses against microbial antigens. The ribotoxins comprise a family of fungal extracellular ribonucleases capable of inactivating ribosomes by specifically cleaving the single phosphodiester linkage at the conserved sarcin/ricin loop of the large rRNA. Subsequent inhibition of protein biosynthesis is followed by apoptosis-induced cell death. Peptides derived from the ribotoxin of *A. fumigatus* modulate immunity in infected mice in a manner consistent with Th1 type responses [67]. An engineered synthetic killer peptide (KP), which functionally mimics fungal killer toxins, binds with β-glucan on fungal cells and mediates direct microbicidal therapeutic effects [132]. Additionally, KP was shown to selectively bind to DCs through MHC-II and CD16/32 and modulate the expression of MHC-II and costimulatory molecules on DCs, thus enhancing their capacity to induce lymphocyte proliferation. Echinocandins, especially caspofungin, have proven potent at variably altering innate immunity against a variety of fungal infections (e.g. *C. parapsilosis*). The hematoregulatory peptide SK&F 107647 is known to elicit a time-dependent increase in $CD11b^+$ MNs and neutrophils in healthy animals [133]. Although administration of SK&F 107647 alone into neutropenic rabbits with disseminated candidiasis did not significantly reduce fungal burden, use of the peptide in combination with low doses of AMB resulted in a significant reduction in lung, liver, spleen, and kidney fungal burdens. Cathelicidin and other cationic peptides, whether constitutively expressed or induced by inflammatory mediators like IL-6 and TNF-α, can modulate cytokine production, alter host gene expression, and minimize inflammation [134-136].

References

[1] Pappagianis D. (1993). The Valley Fever Study Group: Evaluation of the protective efficacy of the killed *Coccidioides immitis* spherule vaccine in humans. *Am. Rev. Respir. Dis.*, 148, 656–60.

[2] Mizutani S, Endo M, Ino-Ue T, Kurasawa M, Uno Y, Saito H, Kato I, Takesako K. (2000). Immunization with the *Candida albicans* membrane fraction and in combination with fluconazole protects against systemic fungal infections. *Antimicrob. Agents Chemother.*, 44, 243–247.

[3] Spellberg B, Ibrahim AS, Lin L, Avanesian V, Fu Y, Lipke P, Otoo H, Ho T, Edwards JE Jr. (2008). Antibody titer threshold predicts anti-candidal vaccine efficacy even though the mechanism of protection is induction of cell-mediated immunity. *J. Infect. Dis.*, 197, 967-971.

[4] Lin L, Ibrahim AS, Avanesian V, Edwards JE Jr, Fu Y, Baquir B, Taub R, Spellberg B. (2008). Considerable differences in vaccine immunogenicities and efficacies related to the diluent used for aluminum hydroxide adjuvant. *Clin. Vaccine Immunol.*, 15, 582-584.

[5] Paulovicová E, Bystrický S, Machová E, Bujdáková H. (2008). Immune responsiveness of a novel peptidoglycan conjugate prepared from surface *Candida* immunogens: mannan and CR3-related protein. *FEMS Immunol. Med. Microbiol.*, 53, 421-428.

[6] Martínez-López R, Nombela C, Diez-Orejas R, Monteoliva L, Gil C. (2008). Immunoproteomic analysis of the protective response obtained from vaccination with *Candida albicans* ecm33 cell wall mutant in mice. *Proteomics*, 8, 2651-2664.

[7] Wu X, Lipinski T, Paszkiewicz E, Bundle DR. (2008). Synthesis and immunochemical characterization of S-linked glycoconjugate vaccines against *Candida albicans*. *Chemistry*, 14, 6474-6482.

[8] Wu X, Lipinski T, Carrel FR, Bailey JJ, Bundle DR. (2007). Synthesis and immunochemical studies on a *Candida albicans* cluster glycoconjugate vaccine. *Org. Biomol. Chem.*, 5, 3477-3485.

[9] Ito JI, Lyons JM, Diaz-Arevalo D, Hong TB, Kalkum M. (2009). Vaccine progress. *Med. Mycol.*, 47, S394-400.

[10] Joel N. Kline. (2007). Eat Dirt CpG DNA and immunomodulation of asthma. *Proc. Am. Thorac. Soc.*, 4, 283–288.

[11] Bozza S, Perruccio K, Montagnoli C, Gaziano R, Bellocchio S, Burchielli E, Nkwanyuo G, Pitzurra L, Velardi A, Romani L. (2003). A

dendritic cell vaccine against invasive aspergillosis in allogeneic hematopoietic transplantation. *Blood*, 102, 3807-3814.

[12] Bozza S, Montagnoli C, Gaziano R, Rossi G, Nkwanyuo G, Bellocchio S, Romani L. (2004). Dendritic cell-based vaccination against opportunistic fungi. *Vaccine*, 22, 857-864.

[13] Bozza S, Gaziano R, Lipford GB, Montagnoli C, Bacci A, Di Francesco P, Kurup VP, Wagner H, Romani L. (2002). Vaccination of mice against invasive aspergillosis with recombinant *Aspergillus* proteins CpG oligodeoxynucleotides as adjuvants. *Microbes Infect*, 4, 1281-1290.

[14] Kinjo T, Miyagi K, Nakamura K, Higa F, Gang X, Miyazato A, Kaku M, Fujita J, Kawakami K. (2007). Adjuvant effect of CpG-oligodeoxynucleotide in anti-fungal chemotherapy against fatal infection with *Cryptococcus neoformans* in mice. *Microbiol. Immunol.*, 51, 741-746.

[15] Ito S, Pedras-Vasconcelos J, Klinman DM. (2005). CpG oligodeoxynucleotides increase the susceptibility of normal mice to infection by *Candida albicans*. *Infect. Immun.*, 73, 6154–6156.

[16] Montagnoli C, Perruccio K, Bozza S, Bonifazi P, Zelante T, De Luca A, Moretti S, D'Angelo C, Bistoni F, Martelli M, Aversa F, Velardi A, Romani L. (2008). Provision of antifungal immunity and concomitant alloantigen tolerization by conditioned dendritic cells in experimental hematopoietic transplantation. *Blood Cells Mol. Dis.*, 40, 55-62.

[17] Zhu F, Ramadan G, Davies B, Margolis DA, Keever-Taylor CA. (2008). Stimulation by means of dendritic cells followed by Epstein-Barr virus-transformed B cells as antigen-presenting cells is more efficient than dendritic cells alone in inducing *Aspergillus* f16-specific cytotoxic T cell responses. *Clin. Exp. Immunol.*, 151, 284-296.

[18] Moll H. (2004). Antigen delivery by dendritic cells. *Int. J. Med. Microbiol.*, 294, 337-344.

[19] Kievit E, Bershad E, Ng E, Sethna P, Dev I, Lawrence TS, Rehemtulla A. (1999). Superiority of yeast over bacterial cytosine deaminase for enzyme/prodrug gene therapy in colon cancer xenografts. *Cancer Res.*, 59, 1417-1421.

[20] Grem JL. (2000). 5-Fluorouracil: forty-plus and still ticking. A review of its preclinical and clinical development. *Investigational New Drugs*, 18, 299-313.

[21] Mallano A, Zamboni S, Carpinelli G, Santoro F, Flego M, Ascione A, Gellini M, Tombesi M, Podo F, Cianfriglia M. (2008). Generation and characterization of a human single-chain fragment variable (scFv)

antibody against cytosine deaminase from Yeast. *BMC Biotechnol*, 8, 68-78.

[22] Cerundolo V, Silk JD, Masr SHi Salio M. (2009). Harnessing invariant NKT cells in vaccination strategies. *Nat. Rev. Immunol.*, 9, 28-38.

[23] Jagannath C, Lindsey DR, Dhandayuthapani S, Xu Y, Hunter RL Jr, Eissa NT. (2009). Autophagy enhances the efficacy of BCG vaccine by increasing peptide presentation in mouse dendritic cells. *Nature Med.*, 15, 267-276.

[24] Murphy JW. (1992). Cryptococcal immunity and immunization. *Adv. Exp. Med. Biol.*, 319, 225-230.

[25] Torosantucci A, Bromuro C, Chiani P, De Bernardis F, Berti F, Galli C, Norelli F, Bellucci C, Polonelli L, Costantino P, Rappuoli R, Cassone A. (2005). A novel glycol-conjugate vaccine against fungal pathogens. *J. Exp. Med.*, 202, 597-606.

[26] Casadevall A, Pirofski LA. (2006). Polysaccharide-containing conjugate vaccines for fungal diseases. *Trends Mol. Med.*, 12, 6-9.

[27] Bellocchio S, Bozza S, Monagnolski C, Perruccio K, Gaziano R, Romani L. (2005). Immunity to *Aspergillus fumigatus*: the basis for immunotherapy and vaccination. *Med. Mycol.*, 43 (Suppl. I), S181-S188.

[28] Romani L, Bistoni F, Gaziano R, Bozza S, Montagnoli C, Perruccio K, Pitzurra L, Bellocchio S, Velardi A, Rasi G, di Francesco P, Garaci E. (2004). Thymosin-α1 activates dendritic cells for antifungal Th1 resistance through Toll-like receptor signaling. *Blood*, 103, 4232-4239.

[29] Lam JS, Mansour MK, Specht CA, Levitz SM. (2005). A model vaccine exploiting fungal mannosylation to increase antigen immunogenicity. *J. Immunol.*, 175, 7496–7503.

[30] Luong M, Lam JS, Chen J, Levitz SM. (2007). Effects of fungal N- and O-linked mannosylation on the immunogenicity of model vaccines. *Vaccine*, 25, 4340-4344.

[31] Abu Elteen K, Hamad M. (2007). Novel antifungal therapies. In Kevin Kavanagh Editor. *New Insights in Medical Mycology* (pp.69-98). Dordrecht: Springer Science and Business Media.

[32] Deepe GS. (1997). Prospects for the development of fungal vaccines. *Clin. Microb. Rev.*, 10, 585-596.

[33] Thomas DP, Viudes A, Monteagudo C, Lazzell AL, Saville SP, López-Ribot JL. (2006). A proteomic-based approach for the identification of *Candida albicans* protein components present in a subunit vaccine that protects against disseminated candidiasis. *Proteomics*, 6, 6033-6041.

[34] Wozniak KL, Ravi S, Macias S, Young ML, Olszewski MA, Steele C, Wormley FL. (2009). Insights into the mechanisms of protective immunity against Cryptococcus neoformans infection using a mouse model of pulmonary cryptococcosis. *PLoS One*, 4(9), e6854.

[35] Specht CA, Nong S, Dan JM, Lee CK, Levitz SM. (2007). Contribution of glycosylation to T cell responses stimulated by recombinant *Cryptococcus neoformans* mannoprotein. *J. Infect. Dis.*, 196, 796-800.

[36] Spellberg BJ, Ibrahim AS, Avanesian V, Fu Y, Myers C, Phan QT, Filler SG, Yeaman MR, Edwards JE Jr. (2006). Efficacy of the anti-Candida rAls3p-N or rAls1p-N vaccines against disseminated and mucosal candidiasis. *J. Infect. Dis.*, 194, 256-260.

[37] Blasi E, Mazzolla R, Barluzzi R, Mosci P, Bistoni F. (1994). Anticryptococcal resistance in the mouse brain: beneficial effects of local administration of heat-inactivated yeast cells. *Infect. Immun.*, 62, 3189-3196.

[38] do Nascimento Martins EM, Reis BS, Fernandes VC, Costa MM, Goes AM, de Andrade AS. (2007). Immunization with radioattenuated yeast cells of *Paracoccidioides brasiliensis* induces a long lasting protection in BALB/c mice. *Vaccine*, 25, 7893-7899.

[39] Marques AF, da Silva MB, Juliano MA, Munhõz JE, Travassos LR, Taborda CP. (2008). Additive effect of P10 immunization and chemotherapy in anergic mice challenged intratracheally with virulent yeasts of *Paracoccidioides brasiliensis*. *Microbes Infect.*, 10, 1251-1258.

[40] Fleuridor R, Lees A, Pirofski L. (2001). A cryptococcal capsular polysaccharide mimotope prolongs the survival of mice with *Cryptococcus neoformans* infection. *J. Immunol.*, 166, 1087–1096.

[41] Pirofski LA. (2001). Polysaccharides, mimotopes and vaccines for fungal and encapsulated pathogens. *Trends Microbio.*, 9, 445–451.

[42] Datta K, Lees A, Pirofski LA. (2008). Therapeutic efficacy of a conjugate vaccine containing a peptide mimotope of cryptococcal capsular polysaccharide glucuronoxylomannan. *Clin. Vaccine Immunol.*, 15, 1176-1187.

[43] Braga CJ, Rittner GM, Muñoz Henao JE, Teixeira AF, Massis LM, Sbrogio-Almeida ME, Taborda CP, Travassos LR, Ferreira LC. (2009). Paracoccidioides brasiliensis vaccine formulations based on the gp43-derived P10 sequence and the Salmonella enterica FliC flagellin. *Infect. Immun.*, 77(4), 1700-1707.

[44] Nakouzi A, Zhang T, Oscarson S, Casadevall A. (2009). The common *Cryptococcus neoformans* glucuronoxylomannan M2 motif elicits non-protective antibodies. *Vaccine*, 27, 3513-3518.

[45] Biondo C, Beninati C, Bombaci M, Messina L, Mancuso G, Midiri A, Galbo R, Teti G. (2003). Induction of T helper type 1 responses by a polysaccharide deacetylase from *Cryptococcus neoformans*. *Infect. Immun.*, 71, 5412–5417.

[46] Dziadek S, Jacques S, Bundle DR. (2008). A novel linker methodology for the synthesis of tailored conjugate vaccines composed of complex carbohydrate antigens and specific TH-cell peptide epitopes. *Chemistry*, 14, 5908-17.

[47] Xin H, Dziadek S, Bundle DR, Cutler JE. (2008). Synthetic glycopeptide vaccines combining beta-mannan and peptide epitopes induce protection against candidiasis. *Proc. Natl. Acad. Sci. USA*, 105, 13526-13531.

[48] Capilla J, Clemons KV, Liu M, Levine HB, Stevens DA. (2009). *Saccharomyces cerevisiae* as a vaccine against coccidioidomycosis. *Vaccine*, 27, 3662-3668.

[49] Cassone A, Torosantucci A. (2006). Opportunistic fungi and fungal infections: the challenge of a single, general antifungal vaccine. *Expert Rev. Vaccines*, 5, 859-867.

[50] Torosantucci A, Bromuro C, Chiani P, De Bernardis F, Berti F, Galli C, Norelli F, Bellucci C, Polonelli L, Costantino P, Rappuoli R, Cassone A. (2005). A novel glycol-conjugate vaccine against fungal pathogens. *J. Exp. Med.*, 202, 597-606.

[51] Ibrahim AS, Spellberg BJ, Avanesian V, Fu Y, Edwards JE. (2006). The anti-*Candida* vaccine based on the recombinant N-terminal domain of Als1p is broadly active against disseminated candidiasis. *Infect. Immun.*, 74, 3039–3041.

[52] Ibrahim AS, Spellberg BJ, Avenissian V, Fu Y, Filler SG, Edwards JE. (2005). Vaccination with recombinant N-terminal domain of Als1p improves survival during murine disseminated candidiasis by enhancing cell-mediated, not humoral, immunity. *Infect. Immun.*, 73, 999–1005.

[53] Spellberg B, Ibrahim AS, Yeaman MR, Lin L, Fu Y, Avanesian V, Bayer AS, Filler SG, Lipke P, Otoo H, Edwards JE Jr. (2008). The antifungal vaccine derived from the recombinant N terminus of Als3p protects mice against the bacterium *Staphylococcus aureus*. *Infect. Immun.*, 76, 4574-4580.

[54] Tarcha EJ, Basrur V, Hung CY, Gardner MJ, Cole GT. (2006). Multivalent recombinant protein vaccine against coccidioidomycosis. *Infect. Immun.*, 74, 5802-5813.
[55] Herr RA, Hung CY, Cole GT. (2007). Evaluation of two homologous proline-rich proteins of *Coccidioides posadasii* as candidate vaccines against coccidioidomycosis. *Infect. Immun.*, 75, 5777-5787.
[56] Wüthrich M, Filutowicz HI, Klein BS. (2000). Mutations of the WI-1 gene yield an attenuated *Blastomyces dermatitidis* strain that induces host resistance. *J. Clin. Invest.*, 106, 1381-1389.
[57] Raska M, Belakova J, Horynova M, Krupka M, Novotny J, Sebestova M, Weigl E. (2008). Systemic and mucosal immunization with *Candida albicans* hsp90 elicits hsp90-specific humoral response in vaginal mucosa which is further enhanced during experimental vaginal candidiasis. *Med. Mycol.*, 46, 411-420.
[58] Wang G, Sun M, Fang J, Yang Q, Tong H, Wang L. (2006). Protective immune responses against systemic candidiasis mediated by phage-displayed specific epitope of *Candida albicans* heat shock protein 90 in C57BL/6J mice. *Vaccine*, 24, 6065-6073.
[59] Raska M, Belakova J, Wudattu NK, Kafková L, Růzicková K, Sebestová M, Kolár Z, Weigl E. (2005). Comparison of protective effect of protein and DNA vaccines hsp90 in murine model of systemic candidiasis. *Folia Microbiol.*, 50, 77-82.
[60] de Bastos Ascenço Soares R, Gomez FJ, de Almeida Soares CM, Deepe GS Jr. (2008). Vaccination with heat shock protein 60 induces a protective immune response against experimental *Paracoccidioides brasiliensis* pulmonary infection. *Infect. Immun.*, 76, 4214-4221.
[61] Guimarães AJ, Frases S, Gomez FJ, Zancopé-Oliveira RM, Nosanchuk JD. (2009). Monoclonal antibodies to heat shock protein 60 alter the pathogenesis of *Histoplasma capsulatum*. *Infect. Immun.*, 77(4), 1357-1367.
[62] Saville SP, Lazzell AL, Chaturvedi AK, Monteagudo C, Lopez-Ribot JL. (2009). Efficacy of a genetically engineered *C. albicans* tet-NRG1 strain as an experimental live attenuated vaccine against hematogenously disseminated candidiasis. *Clin. Vaccine Immunol.*, 16, 430-432.
[63] Ito JI, Lyons JM, Hong TB, Tamae D, Liu YK, Wilczynski SP, Kalkum M. (2006). Vaccinations with recombinant variants of *Aspergillus fumigatus* allergen Aspf3 protect mice against invasive aspergillosis. *Infect. Immun.*, 74, 5075–5084.

[64] Denikus N, Orfaniotou F, Wulf G, Lehmann PF, Monod M, Reichard U. (2005). Fungal antigens expressed during invasive aspergillosis. *Infect. Immun.*, 73, 4704-4713.

[65] Banerjee B, Kurup VP, Greenberger PA, Johnson BD, Fink JN. (2001). Cloning and expression of *Aspergillus fumigatus* allergen Asp f 16 mediating both humoral and cell-mediated immunity in allergic bronchopulmonary aspergillosis (ABPA). *Clin. Exp. Allergy*, 31(5), 761-770.

[66] Cenci E, Mencacci A, Bacci A, Bistoni F, Kurup VP, Romani L. (2000). T cell vaccination in mice with pulmonary aspergillosis. *J. Immunol.*, 165, 381-388.

[67] Svirshchevskaya E, Frolova E, Alekseeva L, Kotzareva O, Kurup VP. (2000). Intravenous injection of major and cryptic peptide epitopes of ribotoxin, Asp f 1 inhibits T cell responses induced by crude *Aspergillus fumigatus* antigens in mice. *Peptides*, 21, 1-8.

[68] Ibrahim AS, Spellberg BJ, Avanesian V, Fu Y, Edwards JE. (2006). The anti-*Candida* vaccines based on the recombinant N-terminal domain of A1s1p is broadly active against disseminated candidiasis. *Infect. Immun.*, 74, 3039-3041.

[69] Xue J, Chen X, Selby D, Hung CY, Yu JJ, Cole GT. (2009). A genetically engineered live attenuated vaccine of *Coccidioides posadasii* protects BALB/c mice against coccidioidomycosis. *Infect. Immun.*, 77, 3196-3208.

[70] Rapaka RR, Goetzman ES, Zheng M, Vockley J, McKinley L, Kolls JK, Steele C. (2007). Enhanced defense against *Pneumocystis carinii* mediated by a novel dectin-1 receptor Fc fusion protein. *J. Immunol.*, 178, 3702-3712.

[71] Bowyer P, Denning DW. (2007). Genomic analysis of allergen genes in *Aspergillus spp*: the relevance of genomics to everyday research. *Med Mycol*, 45, 17-26.

[72] Levitz SM, Tabuni A, Wagner R, Kornfeld H, Smail EH. (1992). Binding of unopsonized *Cryptococcus neoformans* by human bronchoalveolar macrophages: inhibition by a large-molecular-size serum component. *J. Infect. Dis.*, 166, 866-873.

[73] Levitz SM, Dupont MP, Smail EH. (1994). Direct activity of human T lymphocytes and Natural Killer cells against *Cryptococcus neoformans*. *Infect. Immun.*, 62, 194-202.

[74] Ramadan G, Davies B, Kurup VP, Keever-Taylor CA. (2005). Generation of Th1 T cell responses directed to a HLA Class II restricted

epitope from the *Aspergillus* f16 allergen. *Clin. Exp. Immunol.*, 139, 257-267.

[75] Ramadan G, Davies B, Kurup VP, Keever-Taylor CA. (2005). Generation of cytotoxic T cell responses directed to human leucocyte antigen Class I restricted epitopes from the *Aspergillus* f16 allergen. *Clin. Exp. Immunol.*, 140, 81-91.

[76] Tramsen L, Koehl U, Tonn T, Latgé JP, Schuster FR, Borkhardt A, Uharek L, Quaritsch R, Beck O, Seifried E, Klingebiel T, Lehrnbecher T. (2009). Clinical-scale generation of human anti-*Aspergillus* T cells for adoptive immunotherapy. *Bone Marrow Transplant*, 43, 13-19.

[77] Lehrnbecher T, Beck O, Koehl U, Tramsen L. (2009). Cultivated anti-*Aspergillus* T(H)1 cells. *Med Mycol*, 47, S170-174.

[78] Wathrich M, Filutowicz HI, Allen HL, Deepe GS, Klein BS. (2007). V beta1+ J beta1.1+/V alpha2+ J alpha49+ CD4+ T cells mediate resistance against infection with *Blastomyces dermatitidis*. *Infect. Immun.*, 75, 193-200.

[79] Hamad M, El-Younis EM, Yasin SR, Abu-Elteen KH. (2009). TCRVβ clonotypic analysis of vaginal T lymphocytes during experimental vaginal candidiasis in the murine system. *Exp. Clin. Sci.*, 8, 190-197.

[80] Allendoerfer R, Magee DM, Deepe GS Jr, Graybill JR. (1993). Transfer of protective immunity in murine histoplasmosis by a CD4+ T-cell clone. *Infect. Immun.*, 61, 714-718.

[81] Ribedly JM, Christensen JP, Branum K, Doherty PC. (2000). Diminished primary and secondary influenza virus-specific $CD8^+$ T-cell responses in CD4-depleted $Ig^{-/-}$ mice. *J. Virol.*, 74, 9762-9765.

[82] Wang JC, Livingstone AM. (2003). Cutting edge: $CD4^+$ T cell help can be essential for primary $CD8^+$ T cell responses in vivo. *J. Immunol.*, 171, 6339-6343.

[83] Lindell DM, Moore TA, McDonald RA, Toews GB, Huffnagle GB. (2005). Generation of antifungal effector $CD8^+$ T cells in the absence of $CD4^+$ T cells during *Cryptococcus neoformans* infection. *J. Immunol.*, 174, 7920-7928.

[84] Zhou Q, Gault RA, Kozel TR, Murphy WJ. (2006). Immunoglobulin with CD40 stimulation and interleukin-2 protects mice from disseminated cryptococcosis. *Infect. Immun.*, 74, 2161-218.

[85] Grigull L, Beilken A, Schmid H, Kirschner P, Sykora KW, Linderkamp C, Donnerstag F, Goudeva L, Heuft HG, Welte K. (2006). Secondary prophylaxis of invasive fungal infections with combination antifungal

therapy and G-CSF-mobilized granulocyte transfusions in three children with hematological malignancies. *Support Care Cancer*, 14, 783-786.
[86] Grigull L, Pulver N, Goudeva L, Sykora KW, Linderkamp C, Beilken A, Seidemann K, Schmid H, Welte K, Heuft HG. (2006). G-CSF mobilized granulocyte transfusions in 32 paediatric patients with neutropenic sepsis. *Support Care Cancer*, 14, 910-916.
[87] Sachs UJ, Reiter A, Walter T, Bein G, Woessmann W. (2006). Safety and efficacy of therapeutic early onset granulocyte transfusions in pediatric patients with neutropenia and severe infections. *Transfusion*, 46, 1909-1914.
[88] Spellberg BJ, Collins M, Avanesian V, Gomez M, Edwards JE Jr, Cogle C, Applebaum D, Fu Y, Ibrahim AS. (2007). Optimization of a myeloid cell transfusion strategy for infected neutropenic hosts. *J. Leukoc. Biol.*, 81, 632-641.
[89] Pagano L, Valentini CG, Fianchi L, Caira M. (2009). The role of neutrophils in the development and outcome of zygomycosis in haematological patients. *Clin. Microbiol. Infect.*, 15 (Suppl 5), 33-36.
[90] Safdar A, Rodriguez GH, Lichtiger B, Dickey BF, Kontoyiannis DP, Freireich EJ, Shpall EJ, Raad II, Kantarjian HM, Champlin RE. (2006). Recombinant interferon gamma-1β immune enhancement in 20 patients with hematologic malignancies and systemic opportunistic infections treated with donor granulocyte transfusions. *Cancer*, 106, 2664-2671.
[91] Seidel MG, Minkov M, Witt V, Matthes-Martin S, Pötschger U, Worel N, Leitner G, Stary J, Gadner H, Peters C. (2009). Granulocyte transfusions in children and young adults: does the dose matter? *J. Pediatr. Hematol. Oncol.*, 31(3), 166-172.
[92] Wilson Savino. (2006). The thymus is a common target organ in infectious diseases. *PLoS Pathogens*, 2, 472-483.
[93] Savino W, Dardenne M, Marche C, Trophylme D, Dupui JM, Pekovic D, Lapointe N, Bach JF. (1986). Thymic epithelium in AIDS: An immunohistologic study. *Am. J. Pathol.*, 122, 302-307.
[94] Sodora DL, Milush JM, Ware F, Wozniakowski A, Montgomery L, McClure HM, Lackner AA, Marthas M, Hirsch V, Johnson RP, Douek DC, Koup RA. (2002). Decreased levels of recent thymic emigrants in peripheral blood of simian immunodeficiency virus-infected macaques correlates with alterations within the thymus. *J. Virol.*, 76, 9981–9990.
[95] Godfraind C, Holmes KV, Coutelier JP. (1995). Thymus involution induced by mouse hepatitis virus A59 in BALB/c mice. *J. Virol.*, 69, 6541–6547.

[96] Ito M, Nishiyama K, Hyodo S, Shigeta S, Ito T. (1985). Weight reduction of thymus and depletion of lymphocytes of T-dependent areas in peripheral lymphoid tissues of mice infected with *Francisella tularensis*. *Infect. Immun.*, 49, 812–818.

[97] Chen W, Kuolee R, Austin JW, Shen H, Che Y, Conlan JW. (2005). Low dose aerosol infection of mice with virulent type A *Francisella tularensis* induces severe thymus atrophy and CD4þCD8þ thymocyte depletion. *Microb. Pathog.*, 39, 189–196.

[98] Ali-Khan Z. (1978). Cellular changes in the lymphoreticular tissues of C57L/J mice infected with *Echinococcus multilocularis* cysts. *Immunology*, 34, 831-839

[99] Riley EM, Dixon JB, Kelly DF, Cox DA. (1985). The immune response to *Echinococcus granulosus*: sequential histological observations of lymphoreticular and connective tissues during early murine infection. *J. Comp. Pathol.*, 95, 93-104.

[100] Savino W, Leite de Moraes MC, Hontebeyrie-Joskowicz M, Dardenne M. (1989). Studies on the thymus in Chagas' disease. I. Changes in the thymic microenvironment in mice acutely infected with *Trypanosoma cruzi*. *Eur. J. Immunol.*, 19, 1727–1733.

[101] Leite de Moraes MC, Hontebeyrie-Joskowicz M, Leboulanger F, Savino W, Dardenne M, Lepault F. (1991). Studies on the thymus in Chagas' disease. II. Thymocyte subset fluctuations in *Trypanosoma cruzi*-infected mice: Relationship to stress. *Scand. J. Immunol.*, 33, 267–275.

[102] Savino W, Leite de Moraes MC, Silva Barbosa SD, Fonseca EC, Cotta de Almeida V, Hontebeyrie-Joscowicz M. (1992). Is the thymus a target organ in infectious diseases? *Mem. Inst. Oswaldo Cruz (Rio de Janeiro)*, 87, 73–78.

[103] Romani L. (2007). Immunity to Fungi. In Kevin Kavanagh Editor. *New Insights in Medical Mycology* (pp. 1-19). Dordrecht: Springer Science and Business Media,

[104] Romani L. (2004). Immunity to fungal infections. *Nat. Rev. Immunol.*, 4, 1–23.

[105] Romani L. (2002). Immunology of invasive candidiasis. In Calderone RA Editor. *Candida* and *Candidiasis* (pp. 223-241). Washington DC: ASM Press.

[106] Romani L, Puccetti P. (2008). Immune regulation and tolerance to fungi in the lungs and skin. *Chem. Immunol. Allergy*, 94, 124-137.

[107] Roilides E, Dignani MC, Anaissie EJ, Rex JH. (1998). The role of immune-reconstitution in the management of refractory opportunistic fungal infections. *Med. Mycol.*, 36, 12–25.

[108] Jiang C, Magee DM, Cox RA. (1999). Construction of a single-chain interleukin-12-expressing retroviral vector and its application in cytokine gene therapy against experimental Coccidioidomycosis. *Infect. Immun.*, 67, 2996–3001.

[109] Ruan S, McKinley L, Zheng M, Rudner X, D'Souza A, Kolls JK, Shellito JE. (2008). Interleukin-12 and host defense against murine *Pneumocystis pneumonia. Infect. Immun.*, 76, 2130-2137.

[110] Zhou Q, Gault RA, Kozel TR, Murphy WJ. (2007). Protection from direct cerebral *Cryptococcus* infection by interferon-dependent activation of microglial cells. *J. Immunol.*, 178, 5753–5761.

[111] Matsuzaki G, Umemura M. (2007). Interleukin-17 as an effector molecule of innate and acquired immunity against infections. *Microbiol. Immunol.*, 51, 1139-1147.

[112] Stark MA, Huo Y, Burcin TL, Morris MA, Olsen TS, and Ley K. (2005). Phagocytosis of apoptotic neutrophils regulates granulopoiesis via IL-23 and IL-17. *Immunity*, 22, 285-294.

[113] Umemura M, Kawabe T, Shudo K, Kidoya H, Fukui M, Asano M, Iwakura Y, Matsuzaki G, Imamura R, and Suda T. (2004). Involvement of IL-17 in Fas ligand-induced inflammation. *Int. Immunol.*, 16, 1099-1108.

[114] Georgopapadakou NH, Walsh TJ. (1996). Antifungal agents: chemotherapeutic targets and immunologic strategies: mini-review. *Antimicrob Agents Chemother*, 40, 279-291.

[115] Chiou CC, Groll AH, Walsh TJ. (2000). New drugs and novel targets for treatment of invasive fungal infections in patients with cancer. *The Oncologist*, 5, 120-135.

[116] Ribaud P, Chastang C, Latge JP, Baffroy-Lafitte L, Parquet N, Devergie A, Espérou H, Espérou H, Sélimi F, Rocha V, Derouin F, Socié G, Gluckman E. (1999). Survival and prognostic factors of invasive aspergillosis after allogneic bone marrow transplantation. *Clin. Infect. Dis.*, 28, 322-330.

[117] Quezada G, Koshkina NV, Zweidler-McKay P, Zhou Z, Kontoyiannis DP, Kleinerman ES. (2008). Intranasal granulocyte-macrophage colony-stimulating factor reduces the *Aspergillus* burden in an immunosuppressed murine model of pulmonary aspergillosis. *Antimicrob. Agents Chemoth*er, 52, 716–718.

[118] Vora S, Purimetla N, Brummer E, Stevens DA. (1998). Activity of voriconazole, a new triazole, combined with neutrophils on monocytes against *Candida albicans*: Effect of granulocyte colony-stimulating factor and granulocyte-monocyte colony stimulating factor. *Antimicrob. Agents Chemother.*, 42, 907-910.

[119] Roilides E, Holmes A, Blake C, Pizzo PA, Walsh TJ. (1993). Impairment of neutrophil fungicidal activity against *Aspergillus fumigatus* in HIV-infected children. *J. Infect. Dis.*, 167, 905-911.

[120] Razonable RR, Henault M, Lee LN, Laethem C, Johnston PA, Watson HL, Paya CV. (2005). Secretion of pro-inflammatory cytokines and chemokines during amphotericin B exposure is mediated by co-activation of toll-like receptors 1 and 2. *Antimicrob. Agents Chemother*, 49, 1617-1621.

[121] Sau K, Mambula SS, Latz E, Henneke P, Golenbock DT, Levitz S. (2003). The antifungal drug amphotericin B promotes inflammatory cytokine release by toll-like receptor- and CD14-dependent mechanisms. *J. Biol. Chem.*, 278, 37561-37568.

[122] Razonable RR, Henault M, Watson HL, Paya CV. (2005). Nystatin induces secretion of interleukin (IL)-1β, IL-8, and tumor necrosis factor alpha by a toll-like receptor-dependent mechanism. *Antimicrob. Agents Chemother.*, 49, 546-3549.

[123] Simitsopoulou M, Roilides E, Likartsis C, Ioannidis J, Orfanou A, Paliogianni F, Walsh TJ. (2007). Expression of immunomodulatory genes in human monocytes induced by voriconazole in the presence of *Aspergillus fumigatus*. *Antimicrob. Agents Chemother.*, 51, 1048–1054.

[124] Casley WL, Ogrodowczyk C, Larocque L, Jaentschke B, LeBlanc-Westwood C, Menzies JA, Whitehouse L, Hefford MA, Aubin RA, Thorn CF, Whitehead AS, Li X. (2007). Cytotoxic doses of ketoconazole affect expression of a subset of hepatic genes. *J. Toxicol. Environ. Health A*, 70, 1946-1955.

[125] Targan SR, Hanauer SB, van Deventer SJ, Mayer L, Present DH, Braakman T, DeWoody KL, Schaible TF, Rutgeerts PJ. (1997). A short-term study of chimeric monoclonal antibody cA2 to tumor necrosis factor alpha for Crohn's disease cA2 Study group. *N. Engl. J. Med.*, 337, 1029-1035.

[126] Weinblatt ME, Kremer JM, Bankhurst AD, Bulpitt KJ, Fleischmann RM, Fox RI, Jackson CG, Lange M, Burge DJ. (1999). A trial of etanercept, a recombinant tumor necrosis factor receptor: Fc fusion

protein, in patients with rheumatoid arthritis receiving methotrexate. *N. Engl. J. Med.*, 340, 253-259.

[127] Saraceno R, Chimenti S. (2008). How to manage infections in the era of biologics? *Dermatol. Ther.*, 21, 180-186.

[128] Graybill JR, Bocanegra R, Najvar LK, Leobenberg D, Luther MF. (1998). Granulocyte colony stimulating factor and azole antifungal therapy in murine aspergillosis: Role of immune suppression. *Antimicrob. Agents Chemother.*, 42, 2467-2473.

[129] Hamad M. (2008). Antifungal immunotherapy and immunomodulation: a double-hitter approach to deal with invasive fungal infections. *Scand. J. Immunol.*, 67, 533–543.

[130] Li W, Fu M, An JG, Xing Y, Zhang P, Zhang X, Wang YC, Li CX, Tian R, Su WJ, Guan HH, Wang G, Gao TW, Han H, Liu YF. (2007). Host defence against *C. albicans* infections in IgH transgenic mice with V(H) derived from a natural anti-keratin antibody. *Cell Microbiol.*, 9, 306-315.

[131] Nascimento RC, EspÃndola NM, Castro RA, Teixeira PA, Loureiro y Penha CV, Lopes-Bezerra LM, Almeida SR. (2008). Passive immunization with monoclonal antibody against a 70-kDa putative adhesion of *Sporothrix schenckii* induces protection in murine sporotrichosis. *Eur. J. Immunol.*, 38, 3080-3089.

[132] Cenci E, Pericolini E, Mencacci A, Conti S, Magliani W, Bistoni F, Polonelli L, Vecchiarelli A. (2006). Modulation of phenotype and function of dendritic cells by a therapeutic synthetic killer peptide. *J. Leukoc. Biol.*, 79, 40-45.

[133] Lyman CA, Gonzalez C, Schneider M, Lee J, Walsh TJ. (1999). Effects of the hematoregulatory peptide SK&F 107647 alone and in combination with amphotericin B against disseminated candidiasis in persistently neutropenic rabbits. *Antimicrob. Agents Chemother.*, 43, 2165–2169.

[134] Bowdish DE, Davidson DJ, Scott MG, Hancock EW. (2005). Immunomodulatory activities of small host defense peptides. *Antimicrob. Agents Chemotherap.*, 49, 1727-1732.

[135] Diamond G, Russell JP, Bevins CL. (1996). Inducible expression of an antibiotic peptide gene in lipopolysaccharide-challenged tracheal epithelial cells. *Proc. Natl. Acad. Sci. USA*, 93, 5156-5160.

[136] Zhang G, Wu H, Ross CR, Minton JE, Blecha F. (2000). Cloning of porcine NRAMP1 and its induction by lipopolysaccharide, tumor necrosis factor alpha, and interleukin-1beta: role of CD14 and mitogen-activated protein kinases. *Infect. Immun.*, 68, 1086-1093.

Chapter 5

IMMUNOTHERAPY: TARGETING THE PATHOGEN

The mainstay treatment of fungal infections relies on the capacity of drugs such as polyenes, azoles, and echinocandins to target the pathogen and block its infectivity, stop or slow its growth, or kill it altogether. The same rationale has been applied in the search for immune molecules that could mimic the action of antifungal drugs minus the limiting side effects associated with chemotherapy. Therefore, great efforts were put into developing and testing monoclonal antibodies (mAbs), antimicrobial peptides (AMPs), signal cascade inhibitors and other immune molecules that could neutralize, block, opsonize, complement-fix, halt the growth or altogether kill fungal pathogens. The term "inhibitory" that could be used to describe this class of agents should pertain not to their effect on the immune response but rather the detrimental effect they have on the pathogen. By definition, such agents mediate their activity in a passive manner (rapid), and do not require competent immunity to be effective (suitable for use in immunocompromised hosts). However, as pathogen-targeting agents, these modalities remain prone, albeit with a twist, to some of the limitations associated with conventional chemotherapy. For example, they are pathogen-specific with very narrower spectrum of activity, especially in the case of mAbs. This limitation can be overcome by the ease with which pathogen-specific mAbs can be designed and the potential to generate mAbs which recognize antigens common to different fungal species. Induction of fungal resistances as another limitation, is by no means unique to pathogen-targeting immunotherapies, it is common among all pathogen- and to some extent host-targeting treatment approaches. The focus therefore should shift from whether an agent can induce resistance to the mechanisms and differential abilities of various therapies in inducing resistance. In other words, the enigma of microbial resistance can only be managed but probably never solved as will be discussed later. Additional problems that may potentially associate with mAbs and AMPs like cross-reactivity, immune responsiveness, and undesirable side effects are not unique to mAbs and AMPs either.

MONOCLONAL ANTIBODIES

Ever since the introduction of plasma cell hybridoma technology in the mid 1970, an astonishingly large number of hybridomas generated against a whole host of antigens from all kinds of species to produce mAbs for use in research, diagnosis and therapy have been developed. The era of therapeutic mAbs has started in the 1990s with the introduction and approval of several mAbs to treat different forms of cancer. Prominent examples include rituximab (rituxan or MabThera), an anti-CD20 on human B cells, was approved by the FDA in 1997 to treat lymphomas, leukemias and some autoimmune diseases. Infliximab (remicade), a TNF-α inhibitor, received FDA approval in 1998 for the treatment of psoriasis, Crohn's disease, ulcerative colitis, and other autoimmune diseases. Following these and similar successes, development of therapeutic mAbs for the treatment of cancers, autoimmunity, allergy and other diseases has picked up considerable speed. The 2006 Pharmaceutical Research and Manufacturers of America report [*www. phrma.org; Medicines in Development 2006*] has indicated that there are about 160 different mAbs in clinical trial or awaiting FDA approval; the number of therapeutic mAbs grew to 192 in 2008. The same outlook was echoed by the World Health Organization in its 2008 report [1], which estimated that more than 20 mAb-based drugs have been approved for marketing and a further 160 are in the pipelines. Though, the scope of mAb-based experimental antifungal therapy as reported by different research groups is considerable and promising, stories of tangible success are rare. Additionally, of the 192 therapeutic mAbs described in the 2008 Medicines in Development Biotechnology report noted above, only one (the anti-HSP90 Mycograb®) is intended to treat fungal infections (candidiasis).

It is now well accepted that Abs are part of the protective immune response against fungal infections. Ever since the 1960s, it has been known that administration of serum Abs can enhance the outcome of antifungal chemotherapy in cryptococcosis [2]. Fungal infections elicit significant Ab responses; the extent to which such Abs confer protection varies depending on their isotype, subisotype, and titer, the presence or absence of nonprotective competing Abs, and the MHC background of the host [3-6]. IgV_H gene usage variations have also been reported to influence the specificity and protective efficacy of Abs [5]. The appeal of mAb immunotherapy partly derives from its potential to accommodate some of the limitations imposed by vaccine. Additionally, it is possible to engineer mAbs with predetermined fine specificity at the isotype/subisotype and complementarily determining region (CDR) levels. It is possible to prepare Ab therapeutic regimens in pure form and mix them with whatever enhancing additives required. It is also possible to administer them in optimal doses via selected routes. Unlike vaccines, therapeutic mAbs provide immediate protection irrespective of the immune status of the host, which makes them good candidates for use in immunocompromised hosts in particular. Based on the fungal molecular component targeted, experimental antifungal mAbs can be classified into those that target cell wall components, cytoplasmic and signaling pathways, and naturally occurring antifungal antibodies (the anti-idiotype class). Interestingly, this classification echoes that of conventional antifungals (see chapter 2).

Antibodies Targeting Cell Wall Components

The development of protective mAbs against *C. albicans* [7, 8] and *C. neoformans* [9-11] has marked the beginning of a fervent search for protective and therapeutic mAbs against common fungal infections. Generation of effective and protective mAbs against fungi relies on the identification of immunogenic fungal antigens. The fungal cell wall contains several molecular structures involved in fungal pathogenesis and virulence. Therefore, like vaccines, the search for protective mAbs against fungi has focused fungal cell wall constituents. mAbs produced against capsular polysaccharide antigens of *C. neoformans* prolonged survival and decreased fungal burden in *C. neoformans*-infected mice [12, 13]. Fungal beta-glucans have been used as potential targets to develop effective conventional and novel antifungal agents such as echinocandins, yeast killer toxins (KT) and protective Abs [14]. Anti-beta-glucan Abs are detectable in sera of healthy humans and mice. When elicited by glucan-based vaccines, they can exert fungicidal protective activity. Additionally, receptors for beta-glucan cell wall KT can induce the synthesis of fungicidal protective Abs in natural and experimental infections. In a recent study, it was demonstrated that sera from a random population of healthy human subjects contained detectable amounts of anti-laminarin Abs, though at levels lower than that of Abs directed at *C. albicans* β-(1,6)-glucan (pustulan), branched β-(1,3/1,6)-glucan (Pool 1), and mannan [15]. The prevalent isotype of anti-laminarin Abs, like all anti-β-glucans, was IgG and the prevalent subisotype was IgG2 [14, 15]. Anti-laminarin (anti-β-glucan) mAbs, were previously shown capable of inhibiting the synthesis of β-glucan on *C. albicans* cells and hence protect against candidiasis [16]. In a subsequent study [17], it was reported that 2G8 was able to reduce brain and liver fungal burden in mice systemically infected with highly virulent, encapsulated strains of *C. neoformans*. 2G8 was able to reduce *C. neoformans* capsule thickness without interfering with protease or phospholipase production. The Ab was capable of opsonizing acapsular, but not encapsulated, forms of *C. neoformans* for further phagocytosis and killing by monocytes and macrophages. An anti-*C. albicans* Ab prepared in chicken egg yolk (anti-CA IgY) significantly reduced adherence of *C. albicans* to cells of the human pharynx carcinoma cell line FaDu in a dose-dependent manner [18]. Treatment with anti-CA IgY Abs reduced fungal burden in tongue lesions and reduced systemic dissemination in mice with oral candidiasis. The protective potential of anti-CA IgY was attributed to its ability to block adhesion of *C. albicans* to host target cells [18]. In a related study [19], a *C. albicans*-specific chicken egg yolk Ab (IgY) was reported to inhibit the growth of both fluconazole-sensitive and fluconazole-resistant strains of *C. albicans*.

An IgG1 mAb (A9) generated against cell wall extracts of *A. fumigatus* was reported to bind with significant affinity to surface peptides on hyphal and yeast forms of *A. fumigatus* and to inhibit hyphal development and reduce spore germination time. A9 was able to protect against murine invasive aspergillosis by reducing fungal burden and enhancing survival rates [20]. Growth of *Fusarium* species was inhibited in the presence of a fusion protein consisting of recombinant chicken-derived single chain Abs specific against *Fusarium* surface antigens [21]. Expression of the fusion protein in transgenic *Arabidopsis thaliana* plants was protective against *F. oxysporum*. Furthermore, administration of mAbs raised against the glucosylceramide (GlcCer) antigen N-2'-hydroxyhexadecanoyl-1-β-D-glucopyranosyl-9-methyl-4,8-sphingadenine of *F. pedrosoi* reduced fungal growth and enhanced phagocytosis and killing of fungal cells by murine macrophages [22]. G15, a human IgM mAb raised in xeno-mice transgenic for human IgM, IgG2 and Igκ chain, which recognizes epitopes on the capsular polysaccharide GXM of *C. neoformans*, was able to prolong the survival of D strain 24067-sensitized mice following challenge with a lethal dose of virulent *C. neoformans* [5]. G5, an anti-*C. albicans* IgA mAb identified from a hybridoma produced by fusing lymphocytes from *C. albicans*-immunized mouse with Sp2/O cells, exhibited potent *in vitro* candidacidal activity and *in vivo* prophylactic activity [23]. An IgM mAb (C7) raised against *C. albicans*–derived protein glycosyl moieties prolonged survival and enhanced macrophage opsonization in *C. albicans*-infected mice [23]. C7 was reported to ably inhibit *C. albicans* germination and adhesion to HEP2 and oral epithelial cells [24]. Passive treatment with Abs against *P. carinii* demonstrated partial protection against Pcp [25]. Additionally, passive treatment with anti-*P. carinii* IgM mAbs (4F11 and its IgG1 switch variant 4F11G1) protected SCID mice against the development of Pcp [26]. 4F11G1, which recognizes multiple epitopes on the surface of *P. carinii* isolates in mice, also recognizes *P. carinii* isolates from humans, rhesus macaques, rats, and ferrets [26, 27]. Experiments carried out on the protective capacity of 4F11G1 and its (Fab')2 derivative in an intranasal immunoprophylaxis SCID mouse model of Pcp have established that Fc-mediated functions of 4F11G1 (complement fixation in particular) are required for maximum effect of these Abs against *P. carinii* especially when administered passively [28]. Treatment with IgG1 or IgG2a (but not IgG2b) mAbs generated against the *H. capsulatum* cell surface protein HSP60 was reported to significantly prolong survival of mice infected with *H. capsulatum* [29]. Treated infected mice showed reduced fungal burden and organ damage, increased production of IL-12, and TNF-α and decreased production of IL-4 and IL-10. Additionally, both mAbs were able to reduce intracellular fungal survival and increase phagolysosomal fusion of macrophages *in vitro*.

Antibodies Targeting Cytoplasmic Components

In addition to cell wall components, fungal cytoplasmic and signaling moieties have been used to generate therapeutic antifungal mAbs. Anti-gp70, a mAb raised against the 70KD intracellular/secreted glycoprotein component of *P. brasiliensis*, was able to abolish lung granulomas in mice infected with *P. brasiliensis* [30]. The molecular chaperon HSP90 and related proteins are perhaps the most promising and extensively explored targets for development of antifungal mAbs. This is because these proteins help to maintain eukaryotic cell viability; they also represent a class of immunodominant antigens that elicit significant Ab responses in animals and humans. One of the heavily studied and talked about HSP90 variant is that which belongs to *Candida* species (the 47KD HSP90). This variant is expressed by typical pathogenic morphotypes of *Candida* species (pseudohyphae and hyphae) during mucosal and systemic candidiasis. In fact, the appearance of anti-HSP90 Abs in humans and animals with invasive candidiasis is closely associated with recovery from infection [8, 31-36]. A human recombinant anti-HSP90 mAb called Efungumab (trade name is Mycograb®, Novartis Pharmaceuticals Corp., UK) was reported to be protective against murine *C. tropicalis* but not *C. albicans*, *C. krusei*, *C. glabrata* or *C. parapsilosis* infections [31, 34, 35, 37, 38]. In a mouse model of invasive candidiasis, combination therapy using Mycograb® and caspofungin resulted in increased susceptibility of *Candida* species to caspofungin, indicative of synergy between the two agents [35]. Combination therapy consisting of Mycograb® and AMB resulted in complete resolution of *C. albicans*, *C. krusei* and *C. glabrata* infections. In mice infected with *C. parapsilosis* however, Mycograb®-AMB combination therapy cleared the liver and spleen but not the kidneys [31, 39]. In a second study using Mycograb® in combination with AMB to treat candidiasis in mice, it was reported that synergy, defined as a significant increase (FET $P < 0.05$) in the number of negative biopsy specimens compared with those obtained using AMB alone, was evident against fluconazole-resistant strains of *C. albicans* (kidney), *C. krusei* (spleen), *C. glabrata* (spleen), and *C. parapsilosis* (liver and spleen) [37]. Hence it was concluded that complete resolution of infection with *C. albicans*, *C. krusei*, or *C. glabrata* is achievable by combining Mycograb® with AMB. Synergy between Mycograb and AMB in human invasive candidiasis was further confirmed using lipid-associated forms of AMB [40]. Combination therapy with Mycograb® plus AMB, caspofungin, or fluconazole against 8 clinical isolates of *C. neoformans* has indicated that Mycograb® efficiently synergizes with AMB against such infections [38].

Anti-Idiotypes

Use of whole or partial anti-idiotypic mAbs that represent internal images of fungal antigens or toxins to treat invasive fungal infections has been tried with some success. Several yeast genera synthesize and export proteins or glycolproteins with toxic effects (killer toxins or KTs) against sensitive yeast species. Yeast KTs recognize and bind to specific KT receptors on the surface of susceptible microorganisms and form ionic channels in the cytoplasmic membrane or inhibit DNA synthesis [41]. Thus, KT producing fungi gain competitive nutrient and niche advantages over sensitive microorganisms. The first yeast killer toxin was described in *S. cerevisiae* in 1963 [42]; this was followed by the identification of toxins produced by *Candida, Cryptococcus,*

Debaryomyces, Hanseniaspora, Hansenula, Kluyveromyces, Ustilago, Pichia, and other fungal genera. For example, KT produced by the fungus *Pichia anomala* is toxic against a wide variety of microorganisms including hyphomycetes, bacteria (*M. tuberculosis*), and important opportunistic pathogens (*C. albicans, Pneumocystis carinii*) [43]. Direct use of KTs as therapeutic agents against fungal infections is of little promise given their potential toxicity to host cells and the fact that they are labile (temperature and pH sensitive) proteins that remain stable inside the host for short periods of time (often few minutes). To put them to good therapeutic use therefore, a number of anti-idiotypic mAbs have been generated against fungal KTs. The rationale being that fungal species sensitive to KT activity circumvent it in the presence of anti-KT (competing Abs) or anti-KT receptors (KTR) on sensitive fungal cells (blocking Abs). Therefore, anti-idiotypic mAbs that neutralize anti-KT or anti-KTR activity release KT (and/or its receptor) allowing KT to become active against pathogenic fungi. An IgM anti-idiotypic mAb generated in mice immunized with the anti-KT mAb (KT4) exhibited potent killing activity against KT-sensitive *C. albicans* strains [44]. A single-chain recombinant anti-idiotype (KT-scFv) acting as a functional internal image of *P. anomala* KT was synthesized and evaluated for its antimicrobial activity using KT-susceptible *C. albicans* as a model pathogen [45]. A killer decapeptide (KP) containing the first three amino acids of the CDR1 region in KT-scFv anti-idiotype light chain has shown strong candidacidal activity *in vitro* [45]. Post-challenge local administration of KP into rats with vaginal candidiasis (initiated by fluconazole-susceptible or -resistant strains of *C. albicans*) resulted in rapid clearance of the infection. Administration of KP into BALB/c mice challenged with lethal intravenous doses of *C. albicans* significantly prolonged survival (>60 days) compared with that in control mice (3-5 days) [45]. An IgG1κ neutralizing mAb raised against the HM-1 KT (hence the name nmAb-KT) produced by yeast *Williopsis saturnus* var. *mrakii* IFO 0895 has been described [46]. This Ab binds to HM-1 at the sequence 41GSTDGK46 and reduces its killing and glucan synthase inhibitory effects. Treatment of neutropenic T cell-depleted allogeneic bone marrow transplant mice with aspergillosis using nmAb-KT prolonged survival, decreased pathology, and significantly inhibited *A. fumigatus* growth and hyphal development in lung tissues [46]. In a subsequent study by the same group [47], it was further confirmed that recombinant anti-idiotypic scFv Abs can exert antifungal growth activity by inhibiting β-1,3-glucan synthase activity. In that, a series of scFv anti-idiotypes were produced from splenocytes of mice immunized with nmAb-KT; tested fragments were able to inhibit the activity of fungal β-1,3-glucan synthase at IC_{50} values inhibitory to *Candida* species growth.

Radioimmunotherapy

Radioimmunotherapy (RIT) uses Abs labeled with radionuclides to deliver radiation hits to target cell. There are two essential criteria upon which the success (efficacy and safety) of RIT depends. The first pertains to the expression, on target cells, of unique antigens that can be specifically recognized and targeted by specific radiolabeled-molecular probes. Abs are favored over other types of molecular probes because of their exquisite antigen-specificity. This feature enables RIT to target intended cell populations expressing the particular antigen with minimal bystander effects. The second criterion concerns the availability of safe radionuclides that can emit tightly-measured lethal radiation hits against intended targets. Several radionuclides are currently available for targeted radiation therapy ranging in half-life from days (Yttrium ^{90}Y, 2.7 days; Iodine ^{131}I, 8 days) to hours (Rhenium ^{188}Re, 16.9 hrs) to minutes (Bismuth ^{213}Bi, 60 min; indium ^{111}In, 7.7 min). RIT was first developed to treat certain forms of human cancer; the first RIT clinical trial was conducted in the mid 1980s to test the safety and efficacy of this approach against human hepatomas [48]. Since then, several RIT-based anti-cancer drugs have been developed and approved. For example, ibritumomab tiuxetan (Zevalin®), an anti-CD20 mAb conjugated to tiuxetan which chelates isotopes like ^{90}Y or ^{111}In, has been granted FDA approval in 2002 to treat B cell non-Hodgkin's lymphoma. Tositumomab (Bexxar®), also an anti-CD20 mAb covalently-linked to ^{131}I, was approved by the FDA in 2003 to treat relapsed follicular lymphomas or those refractory to rituximab (rituxan®) immunotherapy.

With regard to fungal infections, numerous fungal antigens, whether shared by different fungi or unique to one species, set fungi apart from host cells thus providing for a high degree of discrimination in radiation delivery protocols. The availability of a pan-Ab that can recognize an antigen common to a whole class of pathogens is possible (e.g. 18B7 and D6 mAbs) and desirable. Desirable because it eliminates the need for the expensive and time-consuming routine of generating, radio-processing, and optimizing a wide array of pathogen-specific Abs [49, 50]. Optimal affinity of antifungal Abs as delivery vehicles of radiation is of paramount importance for RIT to be effective. By comparing the quantity of delivered radiation dose, biodistribution and killing activity of anti-*C. neoformans* Abs 18B7 (IgG) and 13F1 (IgM), it was evident that 18B7 was far superior to 13F1 in delivering effective radiation killing activity to lung-localized pathogens [51]. Microorganisms including fungi are susceptible to "direct-hit" and "cross-fire" radiation from a number of α and β particle emitters [50, 52]. The α-emitter ^{213}Bi (half-life = 60 min), which delivers radiation in short bursts with short emission track in tissues, can effectively irradiate and kill small and fast-dividing bacterial pathogens (1μm in diameter, <½ hr doubling time) but not large slow-dividing fungi (≥10μm in diameter, 2-3 hr doubling time). Hence, the use of α- plus β-emitters like ^{188}Re (half-life >16 hrs) might be a better choice to effectively and comprehensively irradiate and kill fungal pathogens [50]. Tightly-measured and highly-targeted radiation delivery is very important to minimize radiation damage to radiation-susceptible host cells. While cell-walled bacteria and fungi require several hundred to several thousand gray (Gy) to be lethally irradiated, mammalian cells can be killed by only few Gy [53].

RIT has been tried to treat experimental *C. neoformans* and *H. capsulatum* infections with some success and with only transient side effects [49, 50, 54-57]. The approach developed by Dadachova and co-workers involves the use of organism-specific mAbs radiolabeled with an imaging radionuclide (e.g. ^{99}mTc or ^{111}In) to localize the site of infection [55-58]. This is then followed by the administration of mAbs radiolabeled with particle emitters such as ^{188}Re or ^{90}Y to irradiate detected pathogen-infested sites [49]. While radiation activities of up to 250 μCi were well tolerated by healthy A/JCr mice for ^{213}Bi- or ^{188}Re-labeled 18B7 mAb therapy, radiation activities of up to 150 μCi in *C. neoformans*-infected counterparts produced only transient toxicity with the lungs of treated mice being free of radiation fibrosis [58]. Antifungal RIT was also shown to reduce mortality in high-burden cryptococcal infections without inducing radiation-resistant cells [59]. The mechanism of action of antifungal RIT varies depending on the radiation dose delivered, which ultimately depends on the type of radionucleotide and its delivery vehicle and how close or distant the complex docks on the surface of target cells. In general terms however, RIT involves direct killing and decreased metabolic activity of target cells. Additionally, RIT has been shown to associate with the induction of apoptosis-like cell death and the occurrence of marked changes in the concentration of IL-2, IL-4, IL-10, TNF-α and IFN-γ suggesting some sort of cooperation between RIT and cellular immunity [60].

Antibody-Based Antifungal Drugs

Encouraging developments towards the introduction of therapeutic mAbs to treat fungal infections notwithstanding, data gaps pertinent to the efficacy and safety of the majority of experimental antifungal mAbs are still considerable with the exception of few specific examples. Efficacy of the recombinant human mAb specific for HSP90 Mycograb® (Efungumab) as an adjunctive drug in patients with culture-proven invasive mycosis has been amply demonstrated [37, 38]. A case report describing prospective treatment of fungal sepsis in a critically ill child with Mycograb® in combination with liposomal AMB or caspofungin was reported to be effective and well-tolerated [61]. Currently, the FDA lists Mycograb® as a drug with an orphan designation for the treatment of invasive candidiasis. Omalizumab (Xolair, Genetech, Novartis), a recombinant DNA-derived humanized IgG1k mAb that selectively binds to human IgE, is an approved drug to treat patients with moderate-to-severe allergic asthma that is uncontrollable with corticosteroid therapy. Recently, it was reported that treatment with anti-IgE (omalizumab) of a cystic fibrosis patient with her third exacerbation of allergic bronchopulmonary aspergillosis (ABPA) improved pulmonary symptoms and lung function; outcomes not achievable with antibiotics or corticosteroids (prednisone) alone [62]. A phase I clinical trial that has evaluated the safety and efficacy of the anti-*C. neoformans* capsular polysaccharide mAb (18B7) when used as an adjunctive therapy in HIV patients with prior history of cryptococcal meningitis has yielded encouraging results [63]. In that, serum antigen titers decreased by a median of 2- and 3-fold at weeks 1 and 2 post-infusion respectively. Side effects in subjects receiving a single infusion of 1-2mg/kg body weight of the drug were minor and the serum half-life of the drug was about 53h.

Side Effects Associated with Antibody-Based Therapies

The emergence of mAb therapy has been associated with a variable spectrum of adverse effects resulting from cross reactivity and immune responsiveness as well as complications associated with biological consequences of target-specific Abs. Allergy, infusion-related reactions (hypotension, rigors, fever, shortness of breath, broncho-spasm, chills, and rash), compromised immunity, and gastrointestinal- and cardiovascular-related side effects that range in severity from mild to fatal were all reported in cancer patients who have received Ab therapy [64, 65]. The jury is still out however with regard to side effects that may associate with antifungal mAbs therapy.

Nonetheless, few points are worth considering especially with the potential arrival of more antifungal mAbs and in light of recent developments in antifungal RIT.

Immune responsiveness to the Fc region of foreign Abs and to the Fab region of both foreign and humanized Abs has been a major obstacle in mAb immunotherapy. Approaches to deal with this problem are scarce but some have been tested and, in some instances, proven more effective and less harmful than whole Abs [66]. Chief among these is the development of humanized mAbs or alternative Ab formats lacking the Fc region altogether. In theory, absence of Fc minimizes interspecies related immune reactivity but does little to minimize the risks of appearance of problematic anti-idiotypes within the host. Nonetheless, Ab modalities like Fabs, scFvs, dAbs, mini-bodies and multi-bodies are gaining increasing appeal to replace whole Abs. For instance, the variable sequence of an anti-idiotypic recombinant killer Ab was used to synthesize CDR-related peptides with differential *in vitro* and *in vivo* anti-*C. albicans* activity [66]. Another set of side effects that could potentially associate with mAb therapy arise from complications related to nonimmunological activities of antibodies as they react with cell surface or cytoplasmic proteins within host cells. For instance, cancer patients and patients suffering from autoimmune and inflammatory diseases can be treated with TNF-α inhibitors. However, as TNF-α is an essential component of the innate immune response, blocking its activity associates with increased risk of fungal infections. A recent case of primary cutaneous cryptococcosis in a rheumatoid arthritis patient being treated with the TNF-α inhibitor adalimumab in combination with methotrexate and hydroxychloroquine has been reported [67]. Furthermore, the FDA has announced on September of 2008 that makers of TNF-α blockers [Cimzia (certolizumab pegol), Enbrel (etanercept), Humira (adalimumab), and Remicade (infliximab)] must strengthen existing warnings on the risk of developing fungal infections as a number of patients with invasive infections due to treatment with these drugs have died.

ANTIMICROBIAL PEPTIDES

Most kingdoms of life secret AMPs or host defense peptides as evolutionarily conserved components of the innate immune response. AMPs are potent, broad spectrum biologics with demonstrated ability to kill enveloped viruses, bacteria, mycobacteria, fungi, and transformed and cancerous cells. On average, AMPs are 12-50 amino acids in length with few positively charged residues (arginine, lysine, histidine) interspersed throughout large portions (>50%) of hydrophobic residues. AMPs occur as α-helixes, β-pleated sheets, linear or cyclic structures. Moderately hydrophobic AMPs with a net positive charge adopt an amphipathic arrangement with the hydrophobic and positively-charged faces occurring in opposite orientations across the plasma membrane of target cells. While the majority of AMPs target pathogens at the cell membrane or cytoplasmic levels, hence their classification here as such, some AMPs have the potential to modulate host immunity as discussed previously.

Mechanism(s) of Action

The activity of AMPs against pathogenic fungi is dependent upon their ability to cause membrane disruption and permeabilization, disrupt and block various biochemical processes, or adversely interact with cytoplasmic and nuclear target molecules (figure 5.1). The ability of AMPs to differentially localize across the membrane lipid bilayer and/or translocate into the cytoplasm, are largely responsible for determining their mechanism of action against target cells. For example, using a series of cyclic peptides of variable ring size that were modeled after gramicidin S 10 (GS10), an analogue of GS, it was demonstrated that biological activity correlates with ring size, degree of beta-structure disruption, net charge, hydrophobicity, amphipathicity, and affinity for lipid membranes [68]. Not only is the chemical composition of AMPs responsible for determining their antimicrobial activity but that of membrane lipids of target cells as well. While increasing the hydrophobicity of analogues of the 26-residue amphipathic α-helical AMP D-V13K results in dramatic decrease in antifungal activity against zygomycetes, increased hydrophobicity dramatically increases their antifungal activity against ascomycetes [69]. Additionally, increased hydrophobicity greatly enhances the hemolytic activity of D-V13K analogues against both zygomycetes (by 1569-fold) and ascomycetes (62-fold). Activity of the L-enantiomer of the winter flounder-derived AMP pleurocidin (Ple) is far more potent (up to 16-fold) against bacterial pathogens and less potent (2-fold) against fungi as compared with that of the D-enantiomer [70]. This is possibly due to the fact that while the L-enantiomer is potent at compromising the integrity of negatively charged liposomes (mimics of bacterial membranes), the D-enantiomer is more potent at causing leakage effects in positively charged liposomes (mimics of fungal membranes). Moreover, the capacity of AMPs to translocate into the cytoplasm (via receptor-mediated or zipper type phagocytosis or other internalization mechanisms) and the presence/absence of target molecules to which translocated AMPs can bind, endows them with the unique ability to alter select biochemical or metabolic processes inside target cells.

Studies that have investigated the influence of structural modifications on the activity of AMPs have also shed some light on the mechanism(s) of action of AMPs and the factors influencing these mechanisms. P-113 peptide and the Trp-rich peptide Ac-KWRRWVRWI-NH(2) have strong antifungal activity against yeast pathogens only at low-salt concentrations. However, antifungal activity of the modified Pac-525 peptide (D-Nal-Pac-525) was retained in media with low or high salt concentrations [71]. End-tagging of the kininogen-derived peptides GKHKNKGKKNGKHNGWK (GKH17) and HKHGHGHGKHKNKGKKN (HKH17) with hydrophobic oligopeptide stretches enhanced their *C. albicans* killing activity [72]. Increased tag length and the use of large Trp and Phe (but not aliphatic) amino acid stretches resulted in enhanced cytocidal activity, better peptide binding to artificial phospholipid membranes, and increased capacity to rupture anionic and cholesterol-void liposomes. Tagging was also shown to render the peptides less toxic and more resistant to degradation by human leukocyte elastase, staphylococcal aureolysin and V8 proteinase [72]. Furthermore, decreasing hydrophobicity and/or increasing cationicity of Ple by Arg or Ser amino acid substitutions at the hydrophobic face did not affect antifungal activity but decreased hemolytic activity of Ple [73]. In its native form, the peptide trappin-2 (P2 or pre-elafin) is an endogenous serine protease inhibitor with potent antimicrobial activity against several microbial and fungal pathogens. Similar antimicrobial activity is achievable with trappin-2 A62D/M63L, a trappin-2 variant lacking antiprotease properties, indicating that trappin-2 exerts its antimicrobial activity through mechanisms independent of its intrinsic antiprotease potential [74].

Natural vs Synthetic AMPS

Natural AMPs occur in bacteria (iturin, bacillomycin, syringiotoxins, cepacidines), fungi (echinocandins), insects (cecropins A and B, drosomycin, dermaseptin) and plants (zeamatin, the cyclopeptide alkaloids amphibine H, frangufloline, nummularine) [75]. The mammalian innate immune system also secrets numerous classes of potent AMPs including those of human origin (histatins, α- and β-defensins, HNP peptides, gallinacin, cathelicidin cationic peptides [hCAP-18], LL-37, protegrins, dermcidin), mouse (CRAMP), rabbit origin (CAP18), pig (protegrins and prophenin), and cattle (indolicidin) [75-77]. Evidence for the involvement of AMPs in immunity against fungal infections is considerable. For instance, human beta-defensins (hBDs 2 and 3) are critical components of innate host defenses at different mucosal surfaces. A recent study has indicated that, under the influence of PMNs, *C. albicans*, a model mucosal surface pathogen, can activate the NF-κB/AP-1 signaling pathway in the esophageal cell line OE21 to upregulate the expression of hBDs [78]. Of the hundreds of natural AMPs discovered so far, some 150 peptides have antifungal activity; hence the term antifungal peptides (AFPs) [79, 80]. Furthermore, the list of synthetic and semisynthetic peptides that have been modeled according to naturally occurring ones is already extensive. The recombinant defensin Tfgd1 synthesized from a cDNA cloned from *Trigonella foenum-graecum* was reported to have broad spectrum antifungal activity [81]. D4E1, a synthetic peptide, is active against *Aspergillus* with the 50% lethal dose (LD_{50}) being achieved at a concentration of 2.1-16.8μg/ml [75]. Treatment with the Paracoccidioid gp43 antigen-derived peptide P10 in combination with AMB, fluconazole, ketoconazole, or itraconazole at 2-30 days following intratracheal challenge of adult mice with virulent isolates of *P. brasiliences* resulted in significant additive protective effects [82].

Based on these findings, it was suggested that this treatment protocol can improve the outcome of chemotherapy, shorten its duration, and bring down the high rates of relapse of *P. brasiliences* infections [75]. The synthetic peptide PLD-118 (BAY 10-8888) has demonstrated a dose-dependent antifungal activity in treating fluconazole-resistant oropharyngeal and esophageal candidiasis [83].

Although the spectrum of activity of intravenous caspofungin (one of several derivatives of the semisynthetic lipopeptide pneumocandin; collective name is echinocandins) is focused on *Candida* species (*C. albicans* and *C. glabrata* but not *C. parapsilosis*), other fungi like *Saccharomyces* species, *P. carinii* and *Aspergillus* species are also susceptible to caspofungin activity (table 1) [84, 85]. FDA approval of caspofungin, micafungin, and anidulafungin in the last decade is proof of the promise of synthetic AMPs (or AFPs) in fighting fungal infections.

AMPs Targeting Fungal Cell Membrane

The majority of AMPs kill fungi by membrane permeabilization and pore formation, which compromise membrane integrity and cause cytoplasmic leakage and cell lysis. Minimum inhibitory concentration (MIC) values of the halocidin synthetic peptide analogue di-K19Hc against clinical isolates of *C. albicans* and *Aspergillus* species are <4 and 16 at 8μg/ml respectively [86]. The peptide rapidly (<30s) kills *C. albicans* by binding to cell wall β-(1,3)-glucan with the subsequent formation of ion channels. Fungicidal activity of the synthetic lactoferrin-derived peptide (Lfpep) and the kaliocin-1 peptide against fluconazole- and AMB-resistant *C. albicans* strains is dependent upon their strong membrane-permeabilization potential [87]. KKVVFKVKFKK is a membrane-active peptide (MP) that inhibits the growth of fluconazole-resistant strains of *C. albicans* at concentrations in the range of 2-32μg/ml [88]. Synthetic analogues of the bactericidal domain of the cationic antimicrobial polypeptide CAP37 (19NQGRHFCGGALIHARFVMTAASC-FQ45) have strong fungicidal activity against fluconazole-sensitive and -resistant isolates of *C. albicans* blastoconidia, *C. guilliermondii*, *C. tropicalis*, *C. pseudotropicalis*, *C. parapsilosis*, and *C. dubliniensis* [89]. The chicken egg white-derived, affinity-purified peptide cystatin (CEWC) was able to inhibit the growth of azole-sensitive *C. albicans*, *C. parapsilosis* and *C. tropicalis* (but not *C. glabrata*) isolates at MIC values comparable with those of fluconazole or the human saliva-derived AMP histatin 5 (0.8-3.3 μmol/L) [90]. Cystatin was also fungicidal to azole-resistant *C. albicans* isolates overproducing the multidrug efflux transporters Cdr1p and Cdr2p [90].

The membrane binding, *Hevea brasiliensis*–derived small (4.7KD) cysteine-rich protein hevein was able to inhibit the growth of *C. albicans*, *C. tropicalis* and *C. krusei* at MIC_{80} values of 95, 12 and 190 μg/ml respectively [91]. Growth inhibition potential of hevein against such oral pathogens was also demonstrated by the disk diffusion method. At a concentration of 30μg/ml, hevein was able to cause a Ca^{2+}-dependent aggregation of *C. tropicalis* yeast cells [91]. The histidine-rich glycoprotein (HRG), an abundant and multimodular plasma protein, binds *Candida* cells and induces breaks in the cell wall rather than the cell membrane. This activity was demonstrated by the finding that HRG lyses ergosterol- but not cholesterol-containing liposomes [92]. The ultra-short antimicrobial lipopeptide palmitoyl-lys-ala-DAla-lys was shown to exert detergent-like effects and membranolytic activity against *A. fumigatus in vitro* [93]. *In vivo* studies involving intranasal administration of DsRed-labeled *A. fumigatus* conidia into immunosuppressed

C57BL/6 wild-type mice followed by lipopeptide treatment have demonstrated the potential of the lipopeptide to degrade and clear hyphal forms and residual conidia in infected lungs. Ple, exhibits strong antifungal activity by disrupting the plasma membrane of target fungal cells [73].

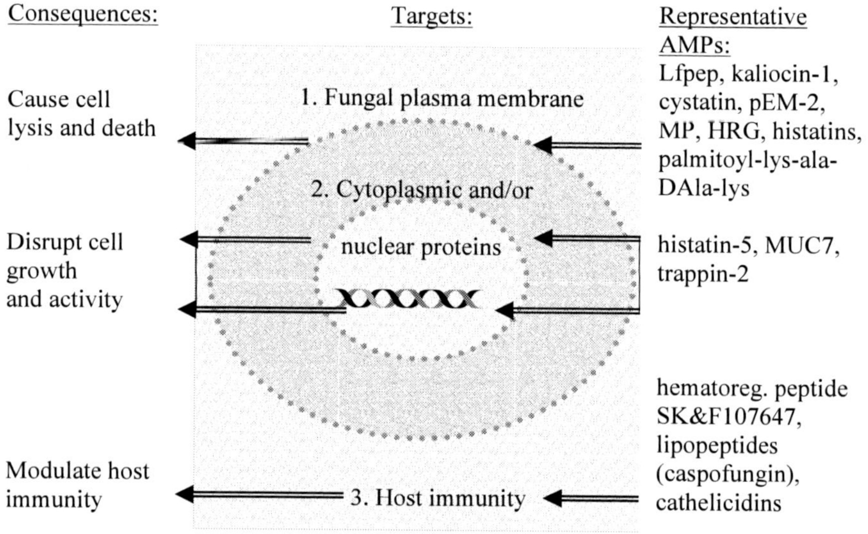

Figure 5.1. Targets and consequences of AMPs with antifungal activity. AMPs target both the pathogen, at the plasma membrane and cytoplasm/nuclear levels, and the host. Depending on the target, which is dictated by peptide molecular composition as well as its cationicity and amphipathicity, the consequences of AMP activities can halt pathogen growth and activity, cause cell lysis and death, or modulate the immune response to better deal with fungal pathogens.

A 13-mer synthetic peptide variant (pEM-2) derived from myotoxin II, a phospholipase A(2) homologue present in *Bothrops asper* snake venom, was shown to exert potent fungicidal activity against pathogenic *Candida* species [94]. Membrane-permeabilization by pEM-2 resulted in 100% killing at a 5μM concentration. The fungicidal effects of piscidin 2 (P2), a striped bass mast cell-derived 22-residue cationic member of the piscidin family of peptides, against human pathogenic fungi was shown to be dependent upon its capacity to cause massive membrane damage and pore formation [95]. Histatins represent a unique family (at least 12 members) of small, cationic, histidine–rich peptides secreted in human saliva by the parotid and submandibular–sublingual glands [96, 97]. Different members of the histatin family can act on fungal plasma membrane or fungal cytoplasmic proteins. Histatins 1 (38 amino acids), 3 (32 amino acids), and 5 (24 amino acids), participate in various biological processes like the formation of enamel pellicle of the teeth, induction of histamine release, inhibition of hemagglutination, inhibition of protease activity and neutralization of lipopolysaccharide [96, 97]. These Histatins exhibit fungicidal activity against several *Candida* species (*C. albicans, C. glabrata* and *C. krusei), S. cerevisiae, C. neoformans* and *A. fumigatus*. They kill or inhibit *Candida* species at near physiological concentrations (15-30μM).

AMPS Targeting the Cytoplasm

While the majority of AMPs kill fungi by compromising the integrity of the plasma membrane, some can inhibit the growth of fungi by interacting with cytoplasmic or nuclear targets to disrupt various intracellular processes [75]. For example, the weak amphipathic structure of histatin-5 enables the peptide to be internalized into the cytoplasm of *C. albicans* cells through receptor-mediated endocytosis or through a translocation transport system in a non-lytic manner. Histatin 5 targets the mitochondria and initiates the loss of transmembrane potential; therefore, inhibition of mitochondrial ATP synthesis protects *C. albicans* against the fungicidal activity of histatin 5 mainly due to reduced accumulation of the peptide [96, 97]. Once internalized, histatin-5 exerts potent candidacidal activities on intracellular targets [98] by, for example, forming free oxygen radicals [99]. *In vitro* studies of the antifungal activity of a cationic peptide derived from the N-terminal portion of human mucin MUC7 peptide (MUC7) against pathogenic *C. albicans* strains has been associated with the upregulation of several glycolytic enzymes within target cells [100]. Trappin-2, an endogenous serine protease inhibitor in neutrophils that controls excess proteolysis during inflammation, exhibits potent antifungal activity against *A. fumigatus* and *C. albicans* at a 5-20μM concentration range [73].

Selective Toxicity of AMPs

The majority of naturally occurring and synthetic AMPs are nonselective; they are toxic to pathogen and host cells alike. However, two aspects of AMP activity are worth considering in this context. First, AMP toxicity is strongly pronounced when used across species; AMPs derived from the same species are much less toxic to host cells. In the case of humans, a large number of human-derived AMPs (histatins, defensins, cathelicidin, etc.) have highly potent antifungal activity against a whole host of fungal pathogens. Therefore, use of human-derived AMPs is one of the possible means by which AMP toxicity can be avoided or at least minimized. Second, some AMPs, irrespective of source species, have specific antifungal selective toxicity owing to factors like host vs pathogen membrane structural variations and the availability (or lack of it thereof) of molecular targets that enable AMPs to mediate their action against specific target cells. For example, IC_{50} of the MP AMP for NIH 3T3 and Jurkat cells is about 100-fold higher than the MIC for *C. albicans* ATCC strain 36232. This suggests that MP is selectively active against fungus but not host cells. Additionally, synthetic non-amphipathic cationic AMPs (CAPs) have been shown to possess selective fungicidal activity against fluconazole-resistant strains of *C. albicans*, *C. tropicalis* and *C. glabrata* in the μM range [101]. The fact that histatins selectively bind to *C. albicans* but not to mammalian cell membranes enables them to express selective candidacidal activity with minimal or no toxic side effects. Substitutions of amino acids that increase the hydrophobicity of cationic AMPs tend to increase antifungal but not anti-host activity [102]. The antifungal activities of the human lactoferrin (hLF)-derived peptide hLF(1-11) and the histatin 5 peptide analogue dhvar5 are comparable to that of AMB against *A. fumigatus* hyphae and conidia [103]. However, whereas hLF(1-11) does not lyse human erythrocytes, dhvar5 at concentrations $\geq$16 μM is hemolytic.

Immunosuppressive Drugs with Antifungal Potential

In theory, immunosuppression is very undesirable as it exacerbates existing infections and increases the susceptibility to opportunistic infections. That unless the action of immunosuppressive drugs against host cells can be replicated in fungal pathogen cells. Immunosuppression can also be of value to counter exuberant inflammatory responses during the course of invasive fungal infections.

Maintenance therapy in transplant patients consists of various regimens of calcineurin inhibitors (CIs) that block T cell activation and inhibit cytokine production (FK506 and CsA), inhibitors of nucleotide synthesis (azathioprine, and mycophenolate mofetil), and inhibitors of intracellular signal transduction (the anti-IL-2 signal blocking and mTOR-targeting agents sirolimus and everolimus). The capacity of certain immunosuppressive agents to interfere with the cellular signaling apparatus of eukaryotic cells has already been explored and utilized as potential antifungal therapy. Calcineurin is a Ca^2/calmodulin-dependent serine/threonine-specific phosphatase that plays a central role in T-cell activation and IL-12 production [104-106]. The macrolide tacrolimus (FK506) and cyclosporine A (CsA) are the two main CIs, hence their wide use to treat solid organ transplant patients. FK506 and CsA can bind with cyclophilin A and the cytosolic protein FK-binding protein 12 (FKBP12), thereby producing drug-protein complexes that inhibit calcineurin activity [107, 108]. Consequently, T cell proliferation, IL-12 production, and ultimately T cell-mediated immunity are inhibited. CIs have been reported to inhibit calcineurin function in the three main human fungal pathogens (*C. albicans*, *C. neoformans*, and *A. fumigatus*) [109-112]. Inhibition of calcineurin activity in *C. albicans* cells results in enhanced susceptibility to azoles, cationic (Ca^{2+}, Na^+, and Li^+) stress, decreased survival in serum and avirulence in systemic murine candidiasis [110, 112]. Further antifungal potential of FK506 and CsA derives from their capacity to interrupt calcineurin-dependent biosynthesis of fungal cell wall 1,3-β-D-glucan contents especially in *A. fumigatus* [113]. This aspect of CIs antifungal activity can enhance the antifungal activity of echinocandins (caspofungin), which block the activity of 1,3-β-D glucan synthase and inhibit 1,3-β-D-glucan synthesis. Therefore, CIs have been used in the past as adjunctive therapies in combination with conventional antifungals [114-116]. Synergism between CIs and fluconazole is attributed to the ability of CIs to enhance the fungicidal activity of fungistatic azoles. Furthermore, CIs are known to enhance fluconazole-mediated inhibition of ergosterol biosynthesis causing massive fungal cell membrane perturbations, hence increasing their own intracellular influx and concentration. The inhibitory effects of FK506 on *C. neoformans* are temperature-dependent; in that *C. neoformans* is resistant to FK506 antifungal activity at 24 °C but not at 37 °C [117]. Although *C. albicans* biofilms are resistant to FK506, CsA or fluconazole in separation, the pathogen is very sensitive to combinations of fluconazole and FK506 or CsA [116]. While *C. albicans* strains lacking FKBP12 or those expressing a dominant FK506-resistant calcineurin mutant subunit (Cnb1-1) are resistant to FK506-fluconazole combinations, they are susceptible to CsA-fluconazole combinations. Lastly, azole-CI combinations have found use as salvage therapies in cases of difficult-to-treat or unresponsive invasive fungal infections [114, 118].

HSP90, the chaperone of molecular chaperones, can influence the path of species evolution by unleashing previously silent genetic variations in response to environmental changes. The remarkable benefits conferred by HSP90 on fungal cells are well manifested in its role of potentiating the evolution of drug resistance through coupling new mutations with immediate phenotypic consequences. The exquisite antifungal activity of HSP90 inhibitors plays on the theme of abrogating the evolution of resistant fungi [119] in response to chemotherapy. The naturally occurring HSP90 inhibitor radicicol (monorden), an inhibitor of Ca^2-signal-dependent cell-cycle regulation in yeast, was reported to minimize the deleterious effects of external $CaCl_2$ influx in *S. cereviciae* by inducing the expression of constitutive active calcineurin [120]. Whether treatment with radicicol could restore calcineurin activity in patients on FK506 or CsA immunosuppressive therapy is yet to be fully addressed.

Despite their desirable immunosuppressive and antifungal activities, treatment with CIs and other biological inhibitors has its limitations. Two such limitations are of interest in the context of this discussion. The fist involves the potential risk of adverse drug-drug interactions between biological inhibitors and azoles (fluconazole in particular) due to potent inhibitory effects of azoles on the mitochondrial P450 enzyme system [121, 122]. The second involves immunosuppression-related susceptibility to opportunistic infections [123-126]. Resistant strains of *C. neoformans* have been isolated from patients with solid organ transplants [123]. FK506 can penetrate the CNS and exacerbates cryptococcal meningitis in rabbits [117]. The nonimmunosuppressive FK506 analogue L-685,818 is also toxic to *C. neoformans in vitro* at 37 °C and is active against FK506-sensitive, but not FK506-resistant, strains of *C. neoformans* [117]. Further work is still needed to establish the full range of antifungal activity of this analogue against invasive and systemic fungal infections. Unlike tacrolimus, the immunosuppressant sirolimus (rapamycin or rapamune), which was first developed as an antifungal drug, inhibits the response to IL-2 instead of calcineurin, thereby blocking activation of T and B cells. Sirolimus binds with FKBP12 and the sirolimus/FKBP12 complex inhibits the mTOR pathway. Since its introduction, sirolimus and related derivatives (everolimus) have proven less likely to render patients susceptible to opportunistic infections [127, 128].

REFERENCES

[1] *The WHO Drug Information publication*, (2002), 22(2), 21.

[2] Gordon MA, Lapa E. (1964). Serum protein enhancement of antibiotic therapy in cryptococcosis. *J. Infect. Dis.*, 114, 373-378.

[3] Casadevall A. (1995). Antibody immunity and invasive fungal infections. *Infect. Immun.*, 63, 4211-4218.

[4] Rivera J, Casadevall A. (2005). Mouse genetic background is a major determinant of isotype-related differences for antibody-mediated protective efficacy against *Cryptococcus neoformans*. *J. Immunol.*, 174, 8017-8026.

[5] Maitta RW, Datta K, Chang Q, Luo RX, Witover B, Subramaniam K, Pirofski LA. (2004). Protective and non-protective human immunoglobulin M monoclonal antibodies to *Cryptococcus neoformans* glucuronoxylomannan manifest different specificites and gene use profiles. *Infect. Immun.*, 72, 4810-4818.

[6] Nussbaum G, Yuan R, Casadevall A, Scharff MD. (1996). Immunoglobulin G3 blocking antibodies to the fungal pathogen *Cryptococcus neoformans*. *J. Exp. Med.*, 183, 1905-1909.

[7] Han Y, Cutler JE. (1995). Antibody response that protects against disseminated candidiasis. *Infect. Immun.*, 63, 2714-2719.

[8] Matthews R, Hodgets S, Burnie J. (1995). Preliminary assessment to of a human recombinant antibody fragment to hsp90 in murine invasive candidiasis. *J. Infect. Dis.*, 171, 1668-1671.

[9] Dromer F, Charreire J, Contrepois A, Carbon C, Yeni P. (1987). Protection of mice against experimental cryptococcosis by anti-*Cryptococcus neoformans* monoclonal antibody. *Infect. Immun.*, 55, 749-752.

[10] Sanford JE, Lupan DM, Schlageter AM, Kozel TR. (1990). Passive immunization against *Cryptococcus neoformans* with an isotype-switch family of monoclonal antibodies reactive with cryptococcal polysaccharides. *Infect. Immun.*, 58, 1919-1923.

[11] Mukherjee J, Scharf MD, Casadevall A. (1992). Protective murine monoclonal antibodies to *Cryptococcus neoformans*. *Infect. Immun.*, 60, 4534-4541.

[12] Mukherjee J, Pirofski IA, Scharf MD, Casadevall A. (1994). Antibody mediated protection in mice with lethal intracerebral *Cryptococcus neoforman* infection. *Proc. Natl. Acad. Sci. USA*, 90, 3636-3640.

[13] Mukherjee J, Nassbaum G, Scharf MD, Casadevall A. (1995). Protective and nonprotective monoclonal antibodies to *Cryptococcus neoformans* originating from one B cell. *J. Exp. Med.*, 181, 405-409.

[14] Magliani W, Conti S, Giovati L, Maffei DL, Polonelli L. (2009). Anti-beta-glucan-like immunoprotective candidacidal anti-idiotypic antibodies. *Front Biosci* 2008; 13:6920-6937.

[15] Chiani P, Bromuro C, Cassone A, Torosantucci A. (2009). Anti-beta-glucan antibodies in healthy human subjects. *Vaccine*, 27, 513-519.

[16] Torosantucci A, Bromuro C, Chiani P, De Bernardis F, Berti F, Galli C, Norelli F, Bellucci C, Polonelli L, Costantino P, Rappuoli R, Cassone A. (2005). A novel glycol-conjugate vaccine against fungal pathogens. *J. Exp. Med.*, 202, 597-606.

[17] Rachini A, Pietrella D, Lupo P, Torosantucci A, Chiani P, Bromuro C, Proietti C, Bistoni F, Cassone A, Vecchiarelli A. (2007). An anti-β-glucan monoclonal antibody inhibits growth and capsule formation of *Cryptococcus neoformans in vitro* and exerts therapeutic, anticryptococcal activity *in vivo*. *Infect. Immun.*, 75, 5085–5094.

[18] Ibrahim el-SM, Rahman AK, Isoda R, Umeda K, Van Sa N, Kodama Y. (2008). *In vitro* and *in vivo* effectiveness of egg yolk antibody against *Candida albicans* (anti-CA IgY). *Vaccine*, 26, 2073-2080.

[19] Wang XZ, Fan B, Liu LG, Hu XY, Li RY, Wei Y, Wan Z, Deng XL. (2008). *In vitro* inhibition of oral *Candida albicans* by chicken egg yolk antibody (IgY). *Mycopathologia*, 165, 381-387.

[20] Ashok K. Chaturvedi AK, Kavishwar A, Shiva Keshava GB, Shukla PK. (2005). Monoclonal immunoglobulin G1 directed against *Aspergillus fumigatus* cell wall glycoprotein protects against experimental murine aspergillosis. *Clin. Diag. Lab. Immunol.*, 12, 1063-1068.

[21] Peschen D, Li HP, Fischer R, Kreuzaler F, Liao YC. (2004). Fusion proteins comprising a *Fusarium*-specific antibody linked to antifungal peptides protect plants against a fungal pathogen. *Nature Biotechnology*, 22, 682-683.

[22] Nimrichter L, Barreto-Bergter E, Mendonca-Filho RR, Kneipp LF, Mazzi MT, Salve P, Farias SE, Wait R, Alviano CS, Rodrigues ML. (2004). A monoclonal antibody to glucosylceramide inhibits the growth of *Fonsecaea pedrosoi* and enhances the antifungal action of mouse macrophages. *Microbes Infect.*, 6, 657-665.

[23] Kacishwar A, Shulka PK. (2006). Candidal activity of a monoclonal antibody that binds with glycosyl moieties of proteins of *Candida albicans*. *Med. Mycol.*, 44, 159-167.

[24] Moragues MD, Omaetxebarria MJ, Elguezabal N, Sevilla MJ, Conti S, Polonelli L, Pontón J. (2003). A monoclonal antibody directed against a *Candida albicans* cell wall mannoproteins exerts three anti-*C. albicans* activities. *Infect. Immun.*, 71, 5273-5279.

[25] Gigliotti F, Hughes WT. (1988). Passive immunoprophylaxis with specific monoclonal antibody confers partial protection against *Pneumocystis carinii* pneumonitis in animal models. *J. Clin. Investig.*, 81, 1666–1668.

[26] Gigliotti F, Haidaris CG, Wright TW, Harmsen AG. (2002). Passive intranasal monoclonal antibody prophylaxis against murine *Pneumocystis carinii* pneumonia. *Infect. Immun.*, 70, 1069–1074.

[27] Wells J, Gigliotti F, Simpson-Haidaris PJ, Haidaris CG. (2004). Epitope mapping of a protective monoclonal antibody against *Pneumocystis carinii* with shared reactivity to *Streptococcus pneumoniae* surface antigen PspA. *Infect. Immun.*, 72, 1548–1556.

[28] Daniela S. Alviano, Anderson J. Franzen, Luiz R. Travassos, Carla Holandino, Sonia Rozental, Regina Ejzemberg, Celuta S. Alviano, and Marcio L. Rodrigues. (2004) Melanin from *Fonsecaea pedrosoi* induces production of human antifungal antibodies and enhances the antimicrobial efficacy of phagocytes. *Infect. Immun.*, 72, 229–237.

[29] Guimarães AJ, Frases S, Gomez FJ, Zancopé-Oliveira RM, Nosanchuk JD. (2009). Monoclonal antibodies to heat shock protein 60 alter the pathogenesis of *Histoplasma capsulatum*. *Infect. Immun.*, 77(4), 1357-1367.

[30] De Mattos Grosso D, de Almeida SR, Mariano M, Lopes JD. (2003). Characterization of gp70 and anti-gp70 monoclonal antibodies in *Paracoccidioide brasilienses* pathogenesis. *Infect. Immun.*, 71, 6534-6542.

[31] Matthews RC, Burnie JP. (2004). Recombinant antibodies: a natural partner in combinatorial antifungal therapy. *Vaccine*, 22, 865-71.

[32] Matthews RC. (1992). *Candida albicans* HSP90: Link between protective and auto immunity. *J. Med. Microbiol.*, 36, 367-370.

[33] Matthews RC. (1994). Pathogenicity determinants of *Candida albicans*: Potential targets for immunotherapy. *Microbiology*, 104, 1505-1511.

[34] Matthews RC, Burnie J. (2001). Antifungal antibodies: A new approach to the treatment of systemic candidiasis. *Curr. Opin. Invest. Drugs*, 2, 472-476.

[35] Hodgetts S, Nooney L, Al-Akeel R, Curry A, Awad S, Matthews R, Burnie J. (2008). Efungumab and caspofungin: pre-clinical data supporting synergy. *J. Antimicrob. Chemother*, 61, 1132-1139.

[36] Rowlands HE, Morris K, Graham C. (2006). Human recombinant antibody against Candida. *Pediatr. Infect. Dis. J.*, 25, 959-960.

[37] Matthews RC, Rigg R, Hodgetts S, Carter T, Chapman C, Gregory C, Illidge C, Burnie J. (2003). Preclinical assessment of the efficacy of Mycograb, a human recombinant antibody against fungal HSP90. *Antimicrob. Agents Chemother.*, 47, 2208–2216.

[38] Nooncy L, Matthews RC, Burnie JP. (2005). Evaluation of Mycograb, amphotericin B, caspofungin, and fluconazole in combination against *Cryptococcus neoformans* by checkerboard and time-kill methodologies. *Diagn Microbiol. Infect. Dis.*, 51, 19-29.

[39] Roilides E, Dignani MC, Anaissie EJ, Rex JH. (1998). The role of immune-reconstitution in the management of refractory opportunistic fungal infections. *Med. Mycol.*, 36, 12–25.

[40] Pachl J, Svoboda P, Jacobs F, Vandewoude K, van der Hoven B, Spronk P, Masterson G, Malbrain M, Aoun M, Garbino J, Takala J, Drgona L, Burnie J, Matthews R. (2006). A randomized, blinded, multicenter trial of lipid-associated amphotericin B alone versus in combination with an antibody-based inhibitor of heat shock protein 90 in patients with invasive candidiasis. *Clin. Infect. Dis.*, 42, 1404-1413.

[41] Magliani W, Conti S, Gerloni M, Bertolotti D, Polonelli L. (1997). Yeast killer systems. *Clin. Microbiol. Rev.*, 10, 369-400.

[42] Bevan E, Makower M. (1963). The physiological basis of the killer-character in yeast. In *Proc Xlth Int Congr Genetics*, Pergamon Press, The Netherlands, I, 203.

[43] Polonelli L, Lorenzini R, De Bernardinis F, Morace G. (1986). Potential therapeutic effect of yeast killer toxin. *Mycopathologia*, 96, 103-107.

[44] Polonelli L, Seguy N, Conti M, Gerloni M, Bertolotti D, Cantelli C, Magliani W, Cailliez JC. (1997). Monoclonal yeast killer toxin-like candidacidal anti-idiotypic antibodies. *Clin. Diag. Lab. Immunol.*, 4, 142-146.

[45] Polonelli L, Magliani W, Conti S, Bracci L, Lozzi L, Neri P, Adriani D, De Bernardis F, Cassone A. (2003). Therapeutic activity of an engineered synthetic killer anti-idiotypic antibody fragment against experimental mucosal and systemic candidiasis. *Infect. Immun.*, 71, 6205- 6212.

[46] Selvakumar D, Zhang QZ, Miyamoto M, Furuichi Y, Komiyama T. (2006). Identification and characterization of a neutralizing monoclonal antibody for the epitope on HM-1 killer toxin. *J. Biochem.*, 139, 399-406.

[47] Selvakumar D, Miyamoto M, Furuichi Y, Komiyama T. (2006). Inhibition of fungal β-1,3-glucan synthase and cell growth by HM-1 killer toxin single-chain anti-idiotypic antibodies. *Antimicrob. Agents Chemother.*, 50, 3090–3097.

[48] Order SE, Stillwagon GB, Klein JL, Leichner PK, Siegelman SS, Fishman EK, Ettinger DS, Haulk T, Kopher K, Finney K. (1985). Iodine 131 antiferritin, a new treatment modality in hepatoma: a Radiation Therapy Oncology Group study. *J. Clin. Oncol.*, 3, 1573-1582.

[49] Dadachova E, Casadevall A. (2009). Radioimmunotherapy of Infectious Diseases. *Semin. Nucl. Med.*, 39, 146-153.

[50] Dadachova E, Casadevall A. (2006). Treatment of infection with radiolabeled antibodies. *Q. J. Nucl. Med. Mol. Imaging*, 50, 193-204.

[51] Dadachova E, Bryan RA, Huang X, Ortiz G, Moadel T, Casadevall A. (2007). Comparative evaluation of capsular polysaccharide-specific IgM and IgG antibodies and F(ab')2 and Fab fragments as delivery vehicles for radioimmunotherapy of fungal infection. *Clin. Cancer Res.*, 13, 5629s-5635s.

[52] Goldenberg DM, Sharkey RM, Udem S, Vagg R, Levine GM, Conte P, Swayne LC, Hansen HJ, Cunniff D, Anton J, Linke MJ, Smulian AG, Walzer PD. (1994). Immunoscintigraphy of *Pneumocystis carinii* pneumonia in AIDS patients. *J. Nucl. Med.*, 35, 1028-1034.

[53] Grieb TA, Forng RY, Stafford RE, Lin J, Almeida J, Bogdansky S, Ronholdt C, Drohan WN, Burgess WH. (2005). Effective use of optimized, high-dose (50 kGy) gamma irradiation for pathogen inactivation of human bone allografts. *Biomaterials*, 26, 2033-2042.

[54] Bozza S, Clavaud C, Giovannini G, Fontaine T, Beauvais A, Sarfati J, D'Angelo C, Perruccio K, Bonifazi P, Zagarella S, Moretti S, Bistoni F, Latgé JP, Romani L. (2009). Immune sensing of *Aspergillus fumigatus* proteins, glycolipids, and polysaccharides and the impact on Th immunity and vaccination. *J. Immunol.*, 183, 2407-2414.

[55] Dadachova E, Nakouzi A, Bryan R, Casadevall A. (2003). Ionizing radiation delivered by specific antibody is therapeutic against a fungal infection. *Proc. Natl. Acad. Sci. USA*, 100, 10942-10947.

[56] Dadachova E, Howell RW, Bryan RA, Frenkel A, Nosanchuk JD, Casadevall A. (2004). Susceptibility of human pathogens *Cryptococcus*

neoformans and *Histoplasma capsulatum* to gamma radiation versus radioimmunotherapy with alpha- and beta emitting radioisotopes. *J. Nucl. Med.*, 45, 313-320.

[57] Martinez LR, Bryan RA, Apostolidis C, Morgenstern A, Casadevall A, Dadachova E. (2006). Antibody-guided alpharadiation effectively damages fungal biofilms. *Antimicrob. Agents Chemother.*, 50, 2132-2136.

[58] Dadachova E, Bryan RA, Frenkel A, Zhang T, Apostolidis C, Nosanchuk JS, Nosanchuk JD, Casadevall A. (2004). Evaluation of acute hematologic and long-term pulmonary toxicities of radioimmunotherapy of *Cryptococcus neoformans* infection in murine models. *Antimicrob. Agents Chemother.*, 48, 1004-1006.

[59] Bryan RA, Jiang Z, Huang X, Morgenstern A, Bruchertseifer F, Sellers R, Casadevall A, Dadachova E. (2009). Radioimmunotherapy is effective against high-inoculum *Cryptococcus neoformans* infection in mice and does not select for radiation-resistant cryptococcal cells. *Antimicrob. Agents Chemother.*, 53, 1679-1682.

[60] Dadachova E, Bryan RA, Apostolidis C, Morgenstern A, Zhang T, Moadel T, Torres M, Huang X, Revskaya E, Casadevall A. (2006). Interaction of radiolabeled antibodies with fungal cells and components of the immune system *in vitro* and during radioimmunotherapy for experimental fungal infection. *J. Infect. Dis.*, 193, 1427-1436.

[61] Sutherland A, Ellis D. (2008). Treatment of a critically ill child with disseminated *Candida glabrata* with a recombinant human antibody specific for fungal heat shock protein 90 and liposomal amphotericin B, caspofungin, and voriconazole. *Pediatr. Crit. Care Med.*, 9, e23-25.

[62] Kanu A, Patel K. (2008). Treatment of allergic bronchopulmonary aspergillosis (ABPA) in CF with anti-IgE antibody (omalizumab). *Pediatr. Pulmonol.*, 43, 1249-1251.

[63] Larsen RA, Pappas PG, Perfect J, Aberg JA, Casadevall A, Cloud GA, James R, Filler S, Dismukes WE. (2005). Phase I evaluation of the safety and pharmacokinetics of murine-derived anticryptococcal antibody 18B7 in subjects with treated cryptococcal meningitis. *Antimicrob. Agents Chemother.*, 49, 952-958.

[64] Chen HX, Cleck JN. (2009). Adverse effects of anticancer agents that target the VEGF pathway. *Nat. Rev. Clin. Oncol.*, 6, 465-477.

[65] Bhatia S, Tykodi SS, Thompson JA. (2009). Treatment of metastatic melanoma: an overview. *Oncology (Williston Park)*, 23, 488-496.

[66] Magliani W, Conti S, Cunha RL, Travassos LR, Polonelli L. (2009). Antibodies as crypts of antiinfective and antitumor peptides. *Curr. Med. Chem.*, 16, 2305-2323.
[67] Wilson ML, Sewell LD, Mowad CM. (2008). Primary cutaneous cryptococcosis during therapy with methotrexate and adalimumab. *J. Drugs Dermatol.*, 7, 53-54.
[68] Jelokhani-Niaraki M, Kondejewski LH, Wheaton LC, Hodges RS. (2009). Effect of ring size on conformation and biological activity of cyclic cationic antimicrobial peptides. *J. Med. Chem.*, 52, 2090-2097.
[69] Jiang Z, Kullberg BJ, van der Lee H, Vasil AI, Hale JD, Mant CT, Hancock RE, Vasil ML, Netea MG, Hodges RS. (2008). Effects of hydrophobicity on the antifungal activity of alpha-helical antimicrobial peptides. *Chem. Biol. Drug Des.*, 72, 483-495.
[70] Lee J, Park C, Park SC, Woo ER, Park Y, Hahm KS, Lee DG. (2009). Cell selectivity-membrane phospholipids relationship of the antimicrobial effects shown by pleurocidin enantiomeric peptides. *J. Pept. Sci.*, 15, 601-606.
[71] Wang CW, Yip BS, Cheng HT, Wang AH, Chen HL, Cheng JW, Lo HJ. (2009). Increased potency of a novel D-beta-naphthylalanine-substituted antimicrobial peptide against fluconazole-resistant fungal pathogens. *FEMS Yeast Res.*, 9, 967-970.
[72] Schmidtchen A, Pasupuleti M, Mörgelin M, Davoudi M, Alenfall J, Chalupka A, Malmsten M. (2009). Boosting antimicrobial peptides by hydrophobic oligopeptide end tags. *J. Biol. Chem.*, 284, 17584-17594.
[73] Sung WS, Lee DG. (2008). Pleurocidin-derived antifungal peptides with selective membrane-disruption effect. *Biochem. Biophys. Res. Commun.*, 369, 858-861.
[74] Baranger K, Zani ML, Chandenier J, Dallet-Choisy S, Moreau T. (2008). The antibacterial and antifungal properties of trappin-2 (pre-elafin) do not depend on its protease inhibitory function. *FEBS J.*, 275, 2008-2020.
[75] De Lucca AJ, Walsh T. (2000). Antifungal peptides: Origin, activity and therapeutic potential. *Rev. Iberoam. Micol.*, 17, 116-120.
[76] Zanetti M. (2004). Cathelicidins, multifunctional peptides of the innate immunity. *J. Leukoc. Biol.*, 75, 39-48.
[77] Bowdish DE, Davidson DJ, Scott MG, Hancock EW. (2005). Immunomodulatory activities of small host defense peptides. *Antimicrob. Agents Chemotherap*, 49, 1727-1732.
[78] Steubesand N, Kiehne K, Brunke G, Pahl R, Reiss K, Herzig KH, Schubert S,Schreiber S, Fölsch UR, Rosenstiel P, Arlt A. (2009). The

expression of the beta-defensins hBD-2 and hBD-3 is differentially regulated by NF-kappaB and MAPK/AP-1 pathways in an *in vitro* model of *Candida* esophagitis. *BMC Immunol.*, 12, 10:36.

[79] Abu Elteen K, Hamad M. (2007). Novel antifungal therapies. In Kevin Kavanagh Editor. *New Insights in Medical Mycology* (pp.69-98). Dordrecht: Springer Science and Business Media.

[80] Hamad M. (2008). Antifungal immunotherapy and immunomodulation: a double-hitter approach to deal with invasive fungal infections. *Scand. J. Immunol.*, 67, 533–543.

[81] Olli S, Kirti PB. (2006). Cloning, characterization and antifungal activity of Tfgdl from *Trigonella foenum-graecum L. J. Biochem. Mol. Biol.*, 39, 278-283.

[82] Marques AF, da Silva MB, Juliano MAP, Travassos LR, Taborda CP. (2006). Peptide immunization as an adjuvant to chemotherapy in mice challenged intratracheally with virulent yeast cells of *Paracoccidioides brasiliensis*. *Antimicrob. Agents Chemother.*, 50, 2814-2819.

[83] Petraitis V, Petraitiene R, Kelaher AM, Sarafandi AA, Sein T, Mickiene D, Bacher J, Groll AH, Walsh TJ. (2004). Efficacy of PLD-118, a novel inhibitor of *Candida* isoleucyl-tRNA synthetase, against experimental oropharyngeal and esophageal candidiasis caused by fluconazole-resistant *C. albicans*. *Antimicrob. Agents Chemother.*, 48, 3959-3967.

[84] Denning DW. (2003). Echinocandin antifungal drugs. *Lancet*, 362, 1142–1151.

[85] Pappas PG, Rex JH, Sobel JD, Filler SG, Dismukes WE, Walsh TJ, Edwards JE; Infectious Diseases Society of America. (2006). Guidelines for treatment of candidiasis. *Clin. Infect. Dis.* 2004; 38:161–189.

[86] Jang WS, Kim HK, Lee KY, Kim SA, Han YS, Lee IH. (2006). Antifungal activity of synthetic peptide derived from halocidin, antimicrobial peptide from the tunicate, *Halocynthia aurantium*. *FEBS Lett.*, 580, 1490-1496.

[87] Viejo-Diaz M, Andres MT, Fierro JF. (2005). Different anti-*candida* activities of two human lactoferrin-derived peptides, Lfpep and kaliocin-1. *Antimicrob. Agents Chemother.*, 49, 2583-2588.

[88] Hong SYU, Oh EJ, Lee KH. (1999). *In vitro* antifungal activity and cytotoxicity of a novel membrane-active peptide. *Antimicrob. Agents Chemother.*, 43, 1704-1707.

[89] Pereira HA, Tsyshevskaya-Hoover I, Hinsley H, Logan S, Nguyen M, Nguyen TT, Pohl J, Wozniak K, Fidel PL Jr. (2009). Candidacidal

activity of synthetic peptides based on the antimicrobial domain of the neutrophil-derived protein, CAP37. *Med. Mycol.*, 22, 1-11.

[90] Kolaczkowska A, Kolaczkowski M, Sokolowska A, Miecznikowska H, Kubiak A, Rolka K, Polanowski A. (2009). The antifungal properties of chicken egg cystatin against *Candida* yeast isolates showing different levels of azole resistance. *Mycoses*, Epub ahead of print, PMID: 19549107.

[91] Kanokwiroon K, Teanpaisan R, Wititsuwannakul D, Hooper AB, Wititsuwannakul R. (2008). Antimicrobial activity of a protein purified from the latex of *Hevea brasiliensis* on oral microorganisms. *Mycoses*, 51, 301-307.

[92] Rydengård V, Shannon O, Lundqvist K, Kacprzyk L, Chalupka A, Olsson AK, Mörgelin M, Jahnen-Dechent W, Malmsten M, Schmidtchen A. (2008). Histidine-rich glycoprotein protects from systemic Candida infection. *PLoS Pathog.*, 4, e1000116.

[93] Vallon-Eberhard A, Makovitzki A, Beauvais A, Latgé JP, Jung S, Shai Y. (2008). Efficient clearance of *Aspergillus fumigatus* in murine lungs by an ultrashort antimicrobial lipopeptide, palmitoyl-lys-ala-DAla-lys. *Antimicrob. Agents Chemother.*, 52, 3118-3126.

[94] Murillo LA, Lan CY, Agabian NM, Larios S, Lomonte B. (2007). Fungicidal activity of a phospholipase-A2-derived synthetic peptide variant against *Candida albicans*. *Rev. Esp. Quimioter*, 20, 330-333.

[95] Sung WS, Lee J, Lee DG. (2008). Fungicidal effect and the mode of action of piscidin 2 derived from hybrid striped bass. *Biochem. Biophys. Res. Commun.*, 371, 551-555.

[96] Tsai H, Bobek LA. (1998). Human salivary histatins: promising anti-fungal therapeutic agents. *Crit. Rev. Oral. Biol. Med.*, 9, 480-97.

[97] Edgerton M, Koshlukova SE. (2000). Salivary histatin 5 and its similarities to the other antimicrobial proteins in human saliva. *Adv Dent Res*, 14, 16-21.

[98] Mochon AB, Liu H. (2008). The antimicrobial peptide histatin-5 causes a spatially restricted disruption on the *Candida albicans* surface, allowing rapid entry of the peptide into the cytoplasm. *PLoS Pathog*, 4, e1000190.

[99] Helmerhorst EJ, Troxler RF, Oppenheim FG. (2001). The human salivary peptide histatin 5 exerts its antifungal activity through the formation of reactive oxygen species. Proc. Natl. Acad. Sci. USA, 98, 14637–14642.

[100] Lis M, Bobek LA. (2008). Proteomic and metabolic characterization of a *Candida albicans* mutant resistant to the antimicrobial peptide MUC7 12-mer. *FEMS Immunol. Med. Microbiol.*, 54, 80-91.

[101] Burrows LL, Stark M, Chan C, Glukhov E, Sinnadurai S, Deber CM. (2006). Activity of novel non-amphipathic cationic antimicrobial peptides against *Candida albicans* species. *J. Antimicrob. Chemother.*, 57, 899-907.

[102] Lee DG, Kim PI, Park Y, Woo ER, Choi CH, Hahm KS. (2002). Design of novel peptide analogs with potent fungicidal activity based on PMAP-23 antimicrobial peptide isolated form procine myeloid. *Biochem. Biophys. Res. Commun.*, 293, 231-238.

[103] Lupetti A, van Dissel JT, Brouwer CP, Nibbering PH. (2008). Human antimicrobial peptides' antifungal activity against *Aspergillus fumigatus*. *Eur. J. Clin. Microbiol. Infect. Dis.*, 27, 1125-1129.

[104] Clipstone NA, Crabtree GR. (1993). Calcineurin is a key signaling enzyme in T lymphocyte activation and the target of the immunosuppressive drugs cyclosporin A and FK506. *Ann. NY Acad. Sci.*, 696, 20–30.

[105] Clipstone NA, Crabtree GR. (1992). Identification of calcineurin as a key signaling enzyme in T-lymphocyte activation. *Nature*, 357, 695–697.

[106] O'Keefe SJ, Tamura J, Kincaid RL, Tocci MJ, O'Neill EA. (1992). FK-506- and CsA-sensitive activation of the interleukin-2 promotner by calcineurin. *Nature*, 357, 692–694.

[107] Cardenas ME, Muir RS, Breuder T, Heitman J. (1995). Targets of immunophilin-immunosuppressant complexes are distinct highly conserved regions of calcineurin A. *EMBO J.*, 14, 2772–2783.

[108] Hemenway CS, Heitman J. (1999). Calcineurin. Structure, function, and inhibition. *Cell Biochem. Biophys.*, 30, 115–151.

[109] Cruz, MC, Fox DS, Heitman J. (2001). Calcineurin is required for hyphal elongation during mating and haploid fruiting in *Cryptococcus neoformans*. *EMBO J.*, 20, 1020–1032.

[110] Bader T, Bodendorfer B, Schroppel K, Morschhauser J. (2003). Calcineurin is essential for virulence in *Candida albicans*. *Infect. Immun.*, 71, 5344–5354.

[111] Steinbach WJ, Schell WA, Blankenship JR, Onyewu C, Heitman J, Perfect JR. (2004). *In vitro* interactions between antifungals and immunosuppressants against *Aspergillus fumigatus*. *Antimicrob. Agents Chemother.*, 48, 1664–1669.

[112] Blankenship JR, Wormley FL, Boyce MK, Schell WA, Filler SG, Perfect JR, Heitman J. (2003). Calcineurin is essential for *Candida albicans* survival in serum and virulence. *Eukaryot Cell*, 2, 422–430.

[113] Fortwendel JR, Juvvadi PR, Pinchai N, Perfect BZ, Alspaugh JA, Perfect JR, Steinbach WJ. (2009). Differential effects of inhibiting chitin and 1,3-{beta}-D-glucan synthesis in ras and calcineurin mutants of *Aspergillus fumigatus*. *Antimicrob. Agents Chemother.*, 53, 476-482.

[114] Sun S, Li Y, Guo Q, Shi C, Yu J, Ma L. (2008). *In vitro* interactions between tacrolimus and azoles against *Candida albicans* determined by different methods. *Antimicrob. Agents Chemother.*, 52, 409-417.

[115] Del Poeta M, Cruz MC, Cardenas ME, Perfect JR, Heitman J. (2000). Synergistic antifungal activities of bafilomycin A(1), fluconazole, and the pneumocandin MK-0991/caspofungin acetate (L-743,873) with calcineurin inhibitors FK506 and L-685,818 against *Cryptococcus neoformans*. *Antimicrob. Agents Chemother.*, 44, 739-746.

[116] Uppuluri P, Nett J, Heitman J, Andes D. (2008). Synergistic effect of calcineurin inhibitors and fluconazole against *Candida albicans* biofilms. *Antimicrob. Agents Chemother.*, 52, 1127–1132.

[117] Odom A, Del Poeta M, Perfect J, Heitman J. (1997). The immunosuppressant FK506 and its nonimmunosuppressive analog L-685,818 are toxic to *Cryptococcus neoformans* by inhibition of a common target protein. *Antimicrob. Agents Chemother.*, 41, 156-161.

[118] Candel FJ, Matesanz M, Mensa J. (2008). Sequential prescription of antifungals in invasive fungal infection: the importance of mechanism of action. *Int. J. Antimicrob. Agents*, 32(S2), S133-135.

[119] Cowen LE, Lindquist S. (2005). Hsp90 potentiates the rapid evolution of new traits: drug resistance in diverse fungi. *Science*, 309, 2185-2189.

[120] Chanklan R, Aihara E, Koga S, Takahashi H, Mizunuma M, Miyakawa T. (2008). Inhibition of Ca2+-signal-dependent growth regulation by radicicol in budding yeast. *Biosci. Biotechnol. Biochem.*, 72, 132-138.

[121] Vickers AE, Meyer E, Dannecker R, Keller B, Tynes RE, Maurer G. (1995). Human liver cytochrome P4503A biotransformation of the cyclosporin derivative SDZ IMM 125. *Drug Metab. Dispos*, 23, 321-326.

[122] Kuypers DR. (2009). Immunotherapy in elderly transplant recipients: a guide to clinically significant drug interactions. *Drugs Aging*, 26, 715-737.

[123] Chang HH, Lee NY, Ko WC, Lee HC, Yang YH, Wu CJ, Chang CM. (2009). Voriconazole inhibition of tacrolimus metabolism in a kidney

transplant recipient with fluconazole-resistant cryptococcal meningitis. *Int J. Infect. Dis.*, [Epub ahead of print].

[124] Parekh K, Trulock E, Patterson GA. (2004). Use of cyclosporine in lung transplantation. *Transplant Proc.*, 36, 318S-322S.

[125] Davis JA, Horn DL, Marr KA, Fishman JA. (2009). Central nervous system involvement in cryptococcal infection in individuals after solid organ transplantation or with AIDS. *Transpl. Infect. Dis.*, [Epub ahead of print].

[126] Martín-Dávila P, Blanes M, Fortún J. (2007). Immunosuppression and infection in transplant recipients. *Enferm. Infecc. Microbiol. Clin.*, 25, 143-154.

[127] Aires I, Carvalho D, Remédio F, Possante M, Ferreira A, Pinto JR, Nolasco F, Santos JR. (2009). Sirolimus-induced drug fever in a renal transplant patient: a case report. *Transplant Proc.*, 41, 957-958.

[128] Gibelli NE, Tannuri U, Pinho-Apezzato ML, Tannuri AC, Maksoud-Filho JG, Andrade WC, Velhote MC, Santos MM, Ayoub AA, Marques da Silva M. (2009). Sirolimus in pediatric liver transplantation: a single-center experience. *Transplant Proc.*, 41, 901-903.

Chapter 6

It Has Yet to Deliver!

Despite considerable efforts and resources dedicated towards the development of immune-based antifungal interventions over the last three decades, there has yet to be a single agent approved for clinical use; with the exception of Mycograb® that is. This is in striking contrast with the overwhelming success of immune-based preventive and therapeutic interventions against viral and bacterial infections, cancer, allergy, autoimmunity, and many other disease states. Nothing illustrates this point more than the enormous success of vaccination campaigns that have, for all intents and purposes, wiped out many debilitating diseases caused by viruses and bacteria from polio (Salk and Sabin vaccines) to tuberculosis (Bacillus Calmette-Guérin vaccine). Cancer immunotherapy in the form of mAbs, radioimmunotherapy, cytokine therapy, cell transfer therapy, and vaccines has also moved at a rapid pace in the last 10-15 years (see table 6.1).

Failure to develop antifungal immune-based therapies despite considerable efforts and resources begs the question: why? Several technical and nontechnical problems continue to hinder progress in this area. There is no question that the immense complexity of fungal pathogens and the numerous intricacies and caveats precipitated by pathogen-host interactions are largely to blame in this regard. For example, serious fungal infections occur primarily as secondary consequences to underlying diseases that compromise host immunity. The risk of blunting immunity by vaccination or other forms of immune-based intervention in the immunocompromised limits the number of options that can be used to fight fungal infections. As discussed in chapter 3, fungal infections tend to elicit cellular rather than humoral immune responses, a fact that poses serious limitations on the success of vaccination procedures.

The sophisticated genetic makeup of fungi increases the risk of vaccine-induced pathogen strain replacement.

Table 6.1. Common examples of immunotherapeutic mAbs approved for the treatment of different forms of cancer during the last decade

mAb	*Brand name*	Target antigen	Approved to treat	Date approved
Trastuzumab	*Herceptin*	ErbB2	Breast cancer	1998
Bevacizumab	*Avastin*	Vascular endothelial growth factor	Colorectal cancer	2004
Cetuximab	*Erbitux*	Epidermal growth factor receptor		
Panitumumab	*Vectibix*			2006
Gemtuzumab	*Mylotarg*	CD33	Acute myelogenous leukemia	2000
Rituximab	*Rituxan, Mabthera*	CD20	Non-Hodgkin lymphoma	1997
Ibritumomab	*Zevalin*			2002
Alemtuzumab	*Campath*	CD52	Chronic lymphocytic leukemia	2001

Fungal pathogens, owing to their eukaryotic nature, sophisticated genetic makeup, and ability to switch form endows them with great potential to evade immunity and resist the effects of immunotherapy. Toxic side effects that may associate with immune-based interventions, especially those belonging to the pathogen-targeting immunotherapy (PTI) approach, pose additional and concerns and challenges. Lastly, lumping up the various antifungal immune-based modalities into one block and treating them with the same light is not helping either. It is high time to realize that differences in antifungal immune-based agents and strategies are not mere superficialities but rather entail variable potentialities and distinct limitations. In other words, distinctions have to be made in terms of the exact goal of a specific agent being modulatory (host-targeting immunomodulation or HTI) or therapeutic (PTI) and in terms of the efficacy and safety evaluation approaches employed to test it. This quick survey is by no means comprehensive or exhaustive, but it should give a taste of the kind of technical complexities researchers in the field have to contend with.

In addition to these technical considerations, nontechnical issues such as lack of funding and poor prioritization may have a crippling effect on basic research and applied development in this area. Lack of interest and scarce capital investment on the part of the pharmaceutical industry and the archaic practices of concerned regulatory agencies obviously hinder rather than help efforts to translate laboratory findings into bedside drugs. The tendency to rush to judgment and to raise hopes unjustifiably on the part of the research community is, at the very least, a turn off to the pharmaceutical industry.

MAKING THE DISTINCTION

Lack of clarity and absence of real distinction between different agents and approaches grouped under the broad subject of antifungal immune-based intervention continues to be a source of confusion. Agents and modalities belonging to PTI and HTI have unique mechanism(s) of action and distinct sets of advantages and disadvantages as tentatively summarized in table 6.2. Instead of further examining these issues, the search for fungal vaccines and immunotherapies seems to be going through an empty repetitive cycle. Published literature on the subject has focused, for the most part, on the same organisms, same protocols, same variations (type of adjuvant, type of animal model, route of administration, chemotherapeutic combination to use, etc.), and same means of efficacy evaluation. Focusing on the same set of questions for so long has left other important questions unaddressed and unanswered. This, it seems, is beginning to deplete the field of new concepts and new ideas.

Like chemotherapy, the activity of PTI-derived agents is independent of the immunostatus of the host making them good candidates for use in immunocompromised hosts. But also like chemotherapy, PTI modalities tend to associate with resistance, narrow spectrum of activity, and toxic side effects, though probably at levels considerably less severe than those that associate with chemotherapy. It seems therefore that so long as antifungal therapy continues to target the pathogen, problems that associate with such an approach will persist [1, 2]. In other words, regardless of the source, mechanism of action, chemical composition or delivery system, improvements on chemotherapy or PTI-derived agents can only go so far to partially address some, but not all, of the problems that associate with them. HTI on the other hand presents its own set of promises and problems. By targeting the host, HTI may help avoid or lessen the severity of problems that classically associate with pathogen-targeting therapies (chemical or immunological). But HTI modalities, especially vaccines, require competent immunity to be fully effective.

Table 6.2. Comparative summary of HTI and PTI modalities in terms of mechanism of action, advantages and disadvantages

Class	Mechanism(s) of action	Potential advantages	Potential Disadvantages
Host-targeting immunomodulation (chapter 4)			
Vaccines	Prime the immune response and generate immunologic memory	Minimal toxicity Minimal risk of resistance induction (vaccines may induce pathogen strain replacement) Broad spectrum of activity	Certain modalities (vaccines, mAbs and AMPs) require immunocompetence to be fully effective Cytokine and cell transfer therapies can cause excessive inflammation and tissue injury and inhibit pathogen tolerance
Cytokines and cell transfer therapies	Restore or reshape the balance of prevalent cytokines Reverse the effects of neutropenia Direct killing of pathogens		
mAbs and AMPs	Activate innate and adaptive cellular components, Modulate cytokine synthesis, Modify Th cell differentiation and/or function and alter host cell gene expression		
Pathogen-targeting immunotherapy (chapter 5)			
mAbs	Fungicidal activity mediated by complement- and antibody-dependent cytotoxic reactions and pathogen opsonization Fungistatic-like activities mediated by neutralizing, blocking, and opsonizing antibodies	Passive activity that occurs independent of host immunostatus (rapid and suitable for hosts with compromised immunity) Amenable to design (specificity, dose, and administration route)	Considerable risk of resistance induction Considerable risk of toxic side effects Monoclonal Abs exhibit species-specific (very narrow) spectrum of activity
AMPs	Fungicidal activity mediated by AMPs that permeabilize the cell membrane Fungistatic-like activities mediated by AMPs that disrupt cellular metabolism and those that interrupt cellular signaling cascades		

This, by definition, severely limits the applicability of HTI in host with compromised immunity. Additionally, their use may associate with inflammation, allergy, and accelerated pathogen strain replacement (the equivalent of resistance). Therefore, while the list of agents belonging to antifungal PTI and HTI is extensive, technical and conceptual problems pertinent to efficacy, safety, and resistance continue to delay the introduction of PTI- or HTI-based therapies and control measures.

EFFICACY CONCERNS

Immunocompetence of the host is, by definition, a prerequisite for vaccination to be of any value. However, common opportunistic fungal infections are secondary to compromised immunity precipitated by underlying disease states. In other words, subjects at increased risk of contracting opportunistic infections hardly meet the immunocompetence requirement. Therefore, even if yet-to-be-introduced fungal vaccines succeed in eliciting protective log-lasting immunity in the healthy, those at increased risk will hardly benefit from them! Putative strategies to design vaccines that could stimulate effective immune responses in immunocompromised hosts have been tried [3-5], but the risk of blunting the immune response in such patients persists. A second concern with regard to vaccine efficacy pertains to the fact that the majority of fungal vaccines tested so far tend to elicit Ab-mediated immune responses [6-13]. But as fungal immunity involves, for the most part, adaptive cell-mediated responses as discussed in chapter 3, such vaccination approaches are of limited value. Manipulating the molecular structure of putative vaccines [4, 14, 15], using DCs as fungal antigen delivery systems that could enlist adaptive immunity [16-20], and the inclusion of immunostimulatory adjuvants [3, 21-25] are options that are only beginning to show some promise.

Research work that aims at expanding the goals and scope of fungal vaccines seems to be shaping up as a major quandary. The concept of cross kingdom vaccination and the incessant focus on therapeutic vaccines are two forms in which expanding the goals and scope of vaccination can be realized. But by definition, the goal of vaccination is to generate long lasting pathogen-specific immunologic memory capable of protecting the host against subsequent infections by the same pathogen. Put differently, vaccines are pathogen-specific preventive rather than therapeutic agents. Even cancer vaccines such as the human papilloma virus (HPV) vaccine that is given to young women to prevent the occurrence of cervical cancers and genital warts, are mainly intended to prevent infections that associate with cancer. With regard to cross-kingdom vaccines, experimentation with vaccines protective against immunogenically-related fungal pathogens is becoming fashionable [3, 4, 26-30]. Results obtained thus far suggest that this approach is no more successful than conventional pathogen-specific vaccination procedure. So, unless it is treated as a passing interest, the hype behind this odd phenomenon is rather difficult to understand. For, surely, it is not lack of pathogen-specific immunogenic molecules that is driving this trend. Furthermore, failure to produce effective and safe fungal vaccines by pathogen-specific vaccination methods ought not to be an impetus for further work on this front. This is because the roots of such a failure lie not in the absence of candidate antigens but rather in not adhering to the good old ways of designing and testing fungal vaccines. The issue of prevention vs therapy in the case of fungal vaccines does not seem to arise by design. It is often the case that the efficacy of experimental vaccines is carried out in already infected animals and is evaluated by measuring the capacity of experimental vaccines to clear up existing infections [31-35]. It must be emphasized that, in both of the above cited cases, the squabble is not etymological, vis-à-vis evolution of the term vaccine to carry new or additional meanings. It is rather the bearing of such intellectual exercises on the overall progress of fungal vaccine research. For one thing, procedures and strategies employed to develop and evaluate therapeutic drugs are distinct from those applicable in the case of preventive measures like vaccines. Additionally, trying to develop vaccines with far reaching goals (prevention and treatment) and broad scope (protecting against several pathogens) can hardly be justified considering the total lack of simple monopathogen-specific preventive fungal vaccines despite more than 30 years of work in this area.

The long experience with cell transfer procedures is not free of significant conceptual flaws either. For example, although primary lymphoid organs are subject to numerous infections and infection-related alterations, work on antifungal cell transfer procedures (syngeneic adoptive T cell transfer procedures in particular) has only focused on cells derived from secondary lymphoid organs. But it has long been known that viral [36-38], bacterial [39, 40], fungal [41, 42], and protozoal [43, 44] pathogens infect primary lymphoid organs like the thymus and cause thymic atrophy, depletion of immature $CD4^+CD8^+$ cells, diminished thymocyte proliferation, epithelial network densification, and increased extracellular matrix deposition. One of the potential consequences in such a case is the induction of central tolerance to pathogen-derived antigens [45, 46] and the generation of perturbed T cell repertoires containing autoreactive T cells and/or lacking T cell specificities needed to recognize and handle specific pathogens. Should such a scenario materialize, options to deal with it are limited. Although the introduction of genetically-engineered antigen-specific syngeneic T cells may be entertained as an option, detailed identification of pathogen specific TCRαβ and/or TCRγδ T cell repertoires is required; a task which has already started [47, 48] but yet to be fully explored.

TOXICITY AND SIDE EFFECTS

Toxicity remains a major limiting factor with regard to cytokine, mAb and AMP therapies. For instance, the potential of cytokine therapy to disturb the balance between proinflammatory and anti-inflammatory responses which could lead to adverse consequences (inflammation and tissue damage or pathogen persistence and allergy) is a major concern. Vaccination with cell wall polysaccharides that induce IL-10 production could also precipitate similar adverse effects. Immunosuppressants that target proinflammatory cytokines and interfere with normal inflammatory and immune responses can lead to increased incidence of opportunistic infections. Use of TNF-α antagonists like infliximab, adalimumab, and the receptor fusion protein etanercept has been associated with increased risk of bacterial and fungal infections [49-51]. The potential of cytokines like G-CSF to induce immunosuppression and other adverse effects has also been reported with regard to fungal infections [52].

Adverse effects, which range in severity from mild to fatal, like allergy, infusion-related reactions (hypotension, rigors, fever, shortness of breath, broncho-spasm, chills, and rash), compromised immunity, and gastrointestinal- and cardiovascular-related side effects continue to associate with Ab-based immunotherapy in patients with cancer, allergy, and transplantation [53, 54]. Although side effects associated with antifungal mAb therapy are yet to be documented in a systematic manner, few points are worth considering. Immune responsiveness to the Fc region of foreign Abs and to the Fab region of both foreign and humanized Abs remains a major obstacle. While humanized mAbs or Ab formats lacking the Fc region (Fabs, scFvs, dAbs, mini-bodies and multi-bodies) [55] can in theory minimize inter-species related immune reactivity, they can do little to prevent the generation of problematic anti-idiotypes. Another safety concern related to Ab-based immunotherapy has to do with potential complications that could result from the biological action of antibodies as molecules that interact with host-cell derived target molecules. For example, use of TNF-α inhibitors (adalimumab) was reported to induce immunosuppression and susceptibility to fungal infections (cutaneous cryptococcosis) [56].

The majority of naturally occurring and synthetic AMPs are nonselective; they are toxic to pathogen and host cells alike especially when used across species. Although potentially useful approaches to overcome this problem are foreseeable, they are yet to be meaningfully explored. For example, the immune response in humans produces numerous AMPs (histatins, defensins, cathelicidin, etc.) with potent antifungal activity against a whole host of fungal pathogens. In other words, problems associated with AMP nonselectivity can be countered by using human-derived AMPs. Some AMPs, irrespective of source species, have specific antifungal selective toxicity owing to factors like host vs pathogen membrane structural variations and availability of molecular targets that enable them to mediate their action against specific target cells. For example, the IC_{50} of MP for NIH-3T3 and Jurkat cells is about 100-fold higher than the MIC for *C. albicans* ATCC strain 36232. Synthetic non-amphipathic cationic AMPs (CAPs) have also been been shown to possess selective fungicidal activity against fluconazole-resistant strains of *C. albicans*, *C. tropicalis* and *C. glabrata* in the μM range [57]. Histatins selectively bind to *C. albicans* but not mammalian cell membranes, hence their ability to express selective candidacidal activity with minimal toxicity to host cells [58]. Furthermore, amino acid substitutions that increase the hydrophobicity of cationic AMPs were reported to enhance their antifungal, but not anti-host, activity [59].

Resistance and Pathogen-Strain Replacement

In evolutionary terms, chemotherapy-induced pathogenic resistance can be viewed as a response to selective pressures exerted by drugs. Accordingly, some cells of the target pathogen undergo genetic changes that enable them and their progeny to survive at much higher doses of the drug or become totally resistant to it. These cells quickly replace the more drug-susceptible ones leading to the appearance of drug resistant strains.

Development of bacterial and fungal resistance to chemotherapy along this path is common knowledge. Furthermore, as pathogen-targeting agents, PTI-derived modalities can also impose selection pressures on pathogens similar to those imposed by drugs, though probably at lesser severity.

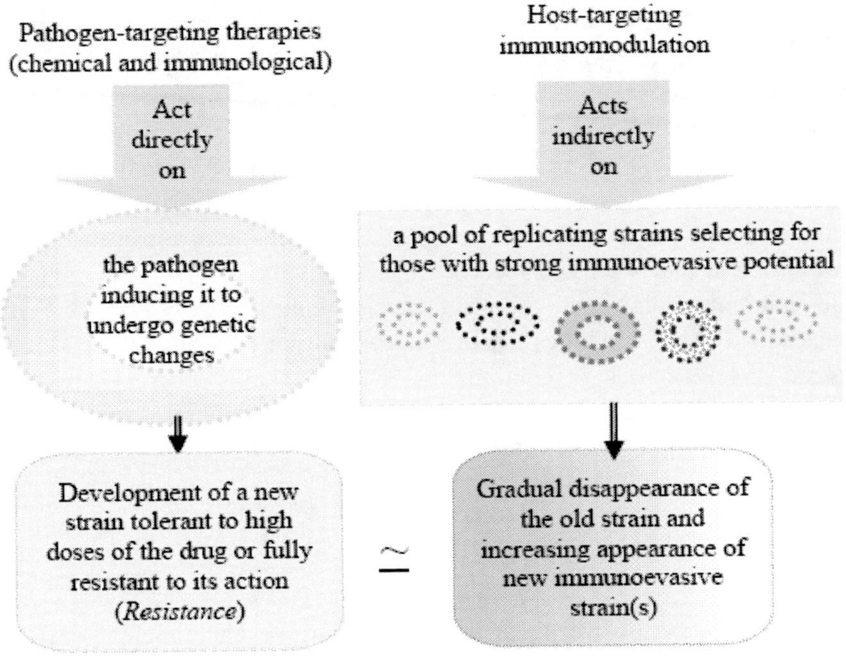

Figure 6.1. Microbial resistance vs pathogen strain replacement. The model proposed here is an attempt to differentiate the general mechanism involved in PTI-induced resistance from that involved in HTI-induced pathogen strain replacement.

What is interesting is that immunity in general and modalities belonging to HTI like vaccines in particular can modify the pattern and pace of pathogen selection. In other words, immunity and vaccination tend to protect the host against a specific pathogenic strain at the risk of opening the door for other more evasive and less susceptible strains to dominate, a phenomenon known as vaccine-induced pathogen strain replacement [60]. Vaccination-related induction of viral and bacterial, but not fungal, resistance has been documented [61-63]. In comparative terms, pathogen-targeting agents (chemotherapy and PTI) induce resistance by directly acting on and manipulating the genetic makeup of the pathogen. Immunity and vaccination on the other hand induce pathogen strain replacement (an equivalent to resistance in effect) by acting on a heterogeneous population of cells and selecting for cells endowed with the ability to endure or evade the immune response (figure 6.1). Therefore, while the immense capacity of fungi to develop resistance to chemotherapy [64-66] predicts that drug-induced resistance occurs in a manner proportional to the genetic complexity of the pathogen [67], it is of little predictive value with regard to the pace and scope of immunity-driven pathogen strain replacement. Interestingly, a study which has surveyed public sequence data of 70 fungal species, has reported that all 70 species contain novel virulence factors with carbohydrate-binding protein effector modules known as LysMs that help to sequester fungal cell wall by-products (chitin oligosaccharides), thereby helping the pathogen to evade immune detection [68]. Therefore, fungal pathogen-strain replacement might be a problem that seems to receive little, if any, attention. Hence, whatever role immunity plays in accelerating the induction of pathogen strain replacement needs to be evaluated. The capacity of HTI modalities to induce fungal pathogen strain replacement, which remains beyond meaningful evaluation at this time as such agents are yet to go into clinical use, is something to be left for the future.

WHAT NOW?

The majority of work carried out so far on experimental antifungal immune-based therapies has focused on addressing the preventive/therapeutic efficacy of a single PTI- or HTI-derived modality at a time. By doing so and without taking into account the overwhelming complexity of fungal infections and the disadvantages that associate with single-modality immune-based therapies, this approach seems to be missing the point. In other words, use of single-modality immune-based therapies misses on the potential complementary power that could result by combining these two distinct approaches. Moreover, studies that have considered combination therapies have addressed specific immune-based modalities in combination with conventional chemotherapy. This is based on the rationale that such combinations can capitalize on the advantages of both approaches. Such an approach, while more promising than *solo* chemotherapy or immunotherapy approaches, is bound to add an additional layer of complexity by bringing to bear the shortcomings of chemotherapy and immune-based therapies. For instance, given that immunotherapy and chemotherapy have the potential to cause side effects and induce resistance it becomes difficult to sort out the contribution(s) of each therapy to these problems when both are used in combination. Worse yet, while positive synergism has been reported with regard to chemo/immunotherapy combinations [34, 69-71], little is known about negative synergism. In other words, the cumulative effects of chemotherapy and immunotherapy on the induction of resistance and the precipitation of side effects are yet to be addressed. Interestingly, studies which have addressed the efficacy of combinations consisting of chemotherapy plus HTI-modalities (cytokines in particular) have shown great promise in minimizing side effects, reducing resistance and improving the general outcome of treatment [72-78]. Combining pathogen-targeting chemotherapy with cytokine or cell transfer therapies could be key to capitalizing on the distinctive positive features of both approaches (figure 6.2). In other words, as both chemotherapy and HTI use different mechanisms to deal with the infection, as they follow different routes to induce resistance and cause side effects, and as using them in combination permits the application of lowered doses of the agents involved, the general outcome can be improved. In contrast, combinations which use chemotherapy plus PTI-derived modalities (mAbs, AMPs or biological inhibitors) may tend to exacerbate fungal infections as both strategies use similar mechanisms of action and follow similar routes of inducing resistance and causing side effects, even if such combinations permit the use of lowered doses. Put differently, such an approach may result in what could be described as negative synergism. What is surprising in all of this is that studies on combinations consisting of PTI- and HTI-derived modalities are still lacking.

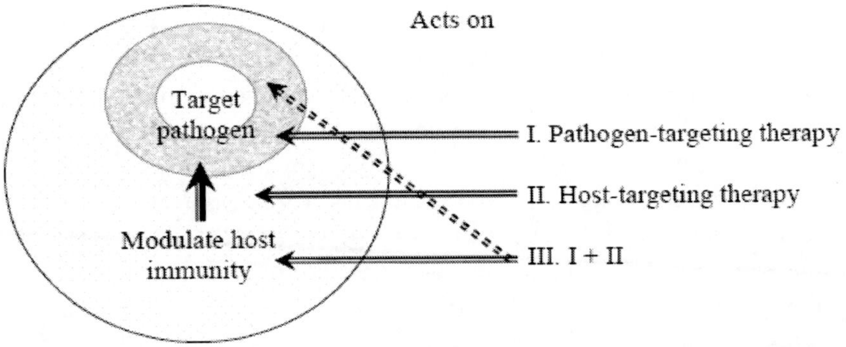

Figure 6.2 Benefits of pathogen- plus host-targeting immunotherapy combinations. While pathogen targeting therapies directly act on the pathogen, host-targeting therapies modulate the immune response of the host to better deal with the pathogen. Although pathogen-targeting therapy applies to both chemotherapy and immunotherapies, it is combinations involving pathogen and host targeting immune-based therapies that are yet to be tested.

To recap, fungi are endowed with an immense potential to evade immunity and resist drug activity. Side effects and resistance are bound to associate with pathogen-targeting therapies (chemotherapy or immunotherapy) and inflammation (and possibly pathogen strain replacement) is bound to associate with HTI. Therefore, it is unlikely for single-modality therapies (chemical or otherwise) to be totally safe and effective. Evolution seems to have come to this conclusion a long time ago; else why the multilayered, multifaceted, and complex antifungal immune response. More than three decades of work on drug-drug or drug-immunotherapy combinations further demonstrates this critical point. Moreover, parallels between fungal immunity and approaches that use combinations of PTI- plus HTI-derived modalities are discernable. For without stating the obvious, fungal immunity involves such a diverse set of innate and adaptive components that modulate immunity (regulatory and helper responses) and target the pathogen (effector responses). Therefore, PTI plus HTI combination therapies may be a suitable approach to approximate the immune response.

On Money and Politics

This is not something scientists and researchers like to think about let alone discuss in scientific publications. In keeping with the same tradition, we will not dwell much on this issue despite the fact that the repercussions of not addressing it can hardly be ignored. Despite the grim statistics and the upward trends in the incidence and mortality of human fungal infections, research in this area is of low priority at many levels. For example, funding for basic and clinical research in the various areas concerned with human fungal infections is "peanuts" compared with what is spent annually on basic and clinical research in areas like cancer, AIDS, diabetes, cardiovascular disease and so on. Capital investment in developing, testing, and translating laboratory bench findings into bedside immunotherapeutics is in no better shape either. Following requests submitted by drug manufacturers, the FDA has designated a number of antifungal drugs as orphan drugs (ODs) (table 6.3). It must be acknowledged here that drug developers and manufacturers understandably brush away the so called orphan diseases (those affecting fewer than 5 individuals per million) as commercially non-feasible areas for capital investment and drug development. Therefore, having a considerable percentage of fungal diseases receiving the orphan disease designation may partially explain the lack of capital investment in developing and commercializing antifungal drugs. This is no truer than in the case of designer antifungals, to which the vast majority of antifungal immunotherapeutics belong.

Table 6.3. List of antifungal products [1] with an FDA Orphan Drug [2] designation

Generic Name (*trade name*)	Designated Indication	Date Designated
AMB lipid complex (*Abelcet)*	Treatment of invasive fungal infections.	1991
AMB inhalation powder	Prevention of pulmonary fungal infections in patients at risk for aspergillosis due to immunosuppressive therapy	2005
Itraconazole suspension	Topical treatment of fungal otitis externa (otomycosis)	2008
Liposomal nystatin *(Nyotran)*	Treatment of invasive fungal infections.	2000
AMB lipid complex (*Abelcet)*	Treatment of invasive coccidioidomycosis, zygomycosis, and candidiasis.	1996
Itraconazole suspension	Topical treatment of fungal otitis externa (otomycosis)	2008
Meclorethamine or nitrogen mustard	Treatment of mycosis fungoides	2004
Methotrexate with laurocapram*Methotrexate (azone)*	Topical treatment of mycosis fungoides.	1990
Nikkomycin Z	Treatment of coccidioidomycosis	2006
Posaconazole (*Posoril)*	Treatment of Zygomycosis	2004
Recomb. Hum. mAb to HSP90 or Efungumab (*Mycograb®)*	Treatment of invasive candidiasis(Currently in phase III clinical trial)	2002
Liposomal AMB*AmBisome*	Treatment of cryptococcal meningitis	1996
Clindamycin (*Cleocin)*	Prevention of *Pneumocystis carinii* pneumonia in AIDS patients.	1988

Source of preliminary data: http://www.fda.gov/downloads/ForIndustry/DevelopingProductsforRareDiseasesConditions/HowtoapplyforOrphanProductDesignation/UCM162066.xls.

[1] Original product list includes more than 2200 drugs.

[2] Orphan Drugs: Products that treat rare disease affecting less than 1 in 200,000 people.

It is worth noting that out of 13 antifungal ODs, only one immunotherapeutic agent was included, namely the recombinant human anti-HSP90 mAb Mycograb®. Current designation of most fungal diseases as ODs notwithstanding, rising trends in fungal infections and the ever growing number of immunocompromised hosts susceptible to opportunistic fungal infections warrant periodic reconsideration.

REFERENCES

[1] Clipstone NA, Crabtree GR. (1993). Calcineurin is a key signaling enzyme in T lymphocyte activation and the target of the immunosuppressive drugs cyclosporin A and FK506. *Ann. NY Acad. Sci.*, 696, 20–30.

[2] Clipstone NA, Crabtree GR. (1992). Identification of calcineurin as a key signaling enzyme in T-lymphocyte activation. *Nature*, 357, 695–697.

[3] Romani L, Kaufmann SH. (1998). Immunity to fungi: editorial overview. *Res. Immunol.*, 149, 277-281.

[4] Bozza S, Perruccio K, Montagnoli C, Gaziano R, Bellocchio S, Burchielli E, Nkwanyuo G, Pitzurra L, Velardi A, Romani L. (2003). A dendritic cell vaccine against invasive aspergillosis in allogeneic hematopoietic transplantation. *Blood*, 102, 3807-3814.

[5] Grem JL. (2000). 5-Fluorouracil: forty-plus and still ticking. A review of its preclinical and clinical development. *Investigational New Drugs*, 18, 299-313.

[6] Romani L, Bistoni F, Gaziano R, Bozza S, Montagnoli C, Perruccio K, Pitzurra L, Bellocchio S, Velardi A, Rasi G, di Francesco P, Garaci E. (2004). Thymosin-α1 activates dendritic cells for antifungal Th1 resistance through Toll-like receptor signaling. *Blood*, 103, 4232-4239.

[7] Lam JS, Mansour MK, Specht CA, Levitz SM. (2005). A model vaccine exploiting fungal mannosylation to increase antigen immunogenicity. *J. Immunol.*, 175, 7496–7503.

[8] Luong M, Lam JS, Chen J, Levitz SM. (2007). Effects of fungal N- and O-linked mannosylation on the immunogenicity of model vaccines. *Vaccine*, 25, 4340-4344.

[9] Joel N. Kline. (2007). Eat Dirt CpG DNA and immunomodulation of asthma. *Proc. Am. Thorac. Soc.*, 4, 283–288.

[10] Bozza S, Montagnoli C, Gaziano R, Rossi G, Nkwanyuo G, Bellocchio S, Romani L. (2004). Dendritic cell-based vaccination against opportunistic fungi. *Vaccine*, 22, 857-864.

[11] Bozza S, Gaziano R, Lipford GB, Montagnoli C, Bacci A, Di Francesco P, Kurup VP, Wagner H, Romani L. (2002). Vaccination of mice against invasive aspergillosis with recombinant *Aspergillus* proteins CpG oligodeoxynucleotides as adjuvants. *Microbes Infect.*, 4, 1281-1290.

[12] Kinjo T, Miyagi K, Nakamura K, Higa F, Gang X, Miyazato A, Kaku M, Fujita J, Kawakami K. (2007). Adjuvant effect of CpG-

oligodeoxynucleotide in anti-fungal chemotherapy against fatal infection with *Cryptococcus neoformans* in mice. *Microbiol. Immunol.*, 51, 741-746.

[13] Ito S, Pedras-Vasconcelos J, Klinman DM. (2005). CpG oligodeoxynucleotides increase the susceptibility of normal mice to infection by *Candida albicans*. *Infect. Immun.*, 73, 6154–6156.

[14] Stumhofer JS, Silver J, Hunter CA. (2007). Negative regulation of Th17 responses. *Semin. Immunol.*, 19, 394-399.

[15] Hunter CA. (2005). New IL-12-family members: IL-23 and IL-27, cytokines with divergent functions. *Nat. Rev. Immunol.*, 5, 521-531.

[16] Roilides E, Dignani MC, Anaissie EJ, Rex JH. (1998). The role of immune-reconstitution in the management of refractory opportunistic fungal infections. *Med. Mycol.*, 36, 12–25.

[17] Bellocchio S, Bozza S, Monagnolski C, Perruccio K, Gaziano R, Romani L. (2005). Immunity to *Aspergillus fumigatus*: the basis for immunotherapy and vaccination. *Med. Mycol.*, 43 (Suppl. I), S181-S188.

[18] Pappagianis D. (1993). The Valley Fever Study Group: Evaluation of the protective efficacy of the killed *Coccidioides immitis* spherule vaccine in humans. *Am. Rev. Respir. Dis.*, 148, 656–60.

[19] Mizutani S, Endo M, Ino-Ue T, Kurasawa M, Uno Y, Saito H, Kato I, Takesako K. (2000). Immunization with the *Candida albicans* membrane fraction and in combination with fluconazole protects against systemic fungal infections. *Antimicrob. Agents Chemother.*, 44, 243–247.

[20] Spellberg B, Ibrahim AS, Lin L, Avanesian V, Fu Y, Lipke P, Otoo H, Ho T, Edwards JE Jr. (2008). Antibody titer threshold predicts anti-candidal vaccine efficacy even though the mechanism of protection is induction of cell-mediated immunity. *J. Infect. Dis.*, 197, 967-971.

[21] Matthews RC. (1992). *Candida albicans* HSP90: Link between protective and auto immunity. *J. Med. Microbiol.*, 36, 367-370.

[22] Wells CA, Salvage-Jones JA, Li X, Hitchens K, Butcher S, Murray RZ, Beckhouse AG, Lo YL, Manzanero S, Cobbold C, Schroder K, Ma B, Orr S, Stewart L, Lebus D, Sobieszczuk P, Hume DA, Stow J, Blanchard H, Ashman RB. (2008). The macrophage-inducible C-type lectin, mincle, is an essential component of the innate immune response to *Candida albicans*. *J. Immunol.*, 180, 7404-7413.

[23] Vázquez-Torres A, Balish E. (1997). Macrophages in resistance to candidiasis. *Microbiol. Mol. Biol. Rev.*, 61, 170-192.

[24] Lin JS, Yang CW, Wang DW, Wu-Hsieh BA. (2005). Dendritic cells cross-present exogenous fungal antigens to stimulate a protective CD8 T cell response in infection by *Histoplasma capsulatum*. *J. Immunol.*, 174, 6282–6291.

[25] Kawai T, Akira S. (2005). Toll-like receptor downstream signaling. *Arthritis. Res. Ther.*, 7, 12-19.

[26] Yauch LE, Mansour MK, Shoham S, Rottman JB, Levitz SM. (2004). Involvement of CD14, toll-like receptors 2 and 4, and MyD88 in the host response to the fungal pathogen *Cryptococcus neoformans in vivo*. *Infect. Immun.*, 72, 5373-5382.

[27] Cerundolo V, Silk JD, Masr SHi Salio M. (2009). Harnessing invariant NKT cells in vaccination strategies. *Nat. Rev. Immunol.*, 9, 28-38.

[28] Jagannath C, Lindsey DR, Dhandayuthapani S, Xu Y, Hunter RL Jr, Eissa NT. (2009). Autophagy enhances the efficacy of BCG vaccine by increasing peptide presentation in mouse dendritic cells. *Nature Med.*, 15, 267-276.

[29] Deepe GS. (1997). Prospects for the development of fungal vaccines. *Clin Microb Rev*, 10, 585-596.

[30] Thomas DP, Viudes A, Monteagudo C, Lazzell AL, Saville SP, López-Ribot JL. (2006). A proteomic-based approach for the identification of *Candida albicans* protein components present in a subunit vaccine that protects against disseminated candidiasis. *Proteomics*, 6, 6033-6041.

[31] Wu X, Lipinski T, Paszkiewicz E, Bundle DR. (2008). Synthesis and immunochemical characterization of S-linked glycoconjugate vaccines against *Candida albicans*. *Chemistry*, 14, 6474-6482.

[32] Wu X, Lipinski T, Carrel FR, Bailey JJ, Bundle DR. (2007). Synthesis and immunochemical studies on a *Candida albicans* cluster glycoconjugate vaccine. *Org. Biomol. Chem.*, 5, 3477-3485.

[33] Murphy JW. (1992). Cryptococcal immunity and immunization. *Adv. Exp. Med. Biol.*, 319, 225-230.

[34] Torosantucci A, Bromuro C, Chiani P, De Bernardis F, Berti F, Galli C, Norelli F, Bellucci C, Polonelli L, Costantino P, Rappuoli R, Cassone A. (2005). A novel glycol-conjugate vaccine against fungal pathogens. *J. Exp. Med.*, 202, 597-606.

[35] Gigliotti F, Hughes WT. (1988). Passive immunoprophylaxis with specific monoclonal antibody confers partial protection against *Pneumocystis carinii* pneumonitis in animal models. *J. Clin. Investig.*, 81, 1666–1668.

[36] De Mattos Grosso D, de Almeida SR, Mariano M, Lopes JD. (2003). Characterization of gp70 and anti-gp70 monoclonal antibodies in *Paracoccidioide brasilienses* pathogenesis. *Infect. Immun.*, 71, 6534-6542.

[37] Matthews RC, Burnie J. (2001). Antifungal antibodies: A new approach to the treatment of systemic candidiasis. *Curr. Opin. Invest. Drugs*, 2, 472-476.

[38] Hodgetts S, Nooney L, Al-Akeel R, Curry A, Awad S, Matthews R, Burnie J. (2008). Efungumab and caspofungin: pre-clinical data supporting synergy. *J. Antimicrob. Chemother.*, 61, 1132-1139.

[39] Rowlands HE, Morris K, Graham C. (2006). Human recombinant antibody against *Candida. Pediatr. Infect. Dis. J.*, 25, 959-960.

[40] Ruth C. Matthews, Gordon Rigg, Samantha Hodgetts, Tracey Carter Caroline Chapman, Carl Gregory, Chris Illidge, and James Burnie. (2003). Preclinical assessment of the efficacy of Mycograb, a human recombinant antibody against fungal HSP90. *Antimicrob. Agents Chemother.*, 47, 2208–2216.

[41] Nooney L, Matthews RC, Burnie JP. (2005). Evaluation of Mycograb, amphotericin B, caspofungin, and fluconazole in combination against *Cryptococcus neoformans* by checkerboard and time-kill methodologies. *Diagn Microbiol. Infect. Dis.*, 51, 19-29.

[42] Magliani W, Conti S, Gerloni M, Bertolotti D, Polonelli L. (1997). Yeast killer systems. *Clin. Microbiol. Rev.*, 10, 369-400.

[43] Bevan E, Makower M. (1963). The physiological basis of the killer-character in yeast. In *Proc XIth Int Congr Genetics*, Pergamon Press, The Netherlands, I, 203.

[44] Polonelli L, Lorenzini R, De Bernardinis F, Morace G. (1986). Potential therapeutic effect of yeast killer toxin. *Mycopathologia*, 96, 103-107.

[45] Polonelli L, Seguy N, Conti M, Gerloni M, Bertolotti D, Cantelli C, Magliani W, Cailliez JC. (1997). Monoclonal yeast killer toxin-like candidacidal anti-idiotypic antibodies. *Clin. Diag Lab. Immunol.*, 4, 142-146.

[46] Polonelli L, Magliani W, Conti S, Bracci L, Lozzi L, Neri P, Adriani D, De Bernardis F, Cassone A. (2003). Therapeutic activity of an engineered synthetic killer anti-idiotypic antibody fragment against experimental mucosal and systemic candidiasis. *Infect. Immun.*, 71, 6205- 6212.

[47] Selvakumar D, Zhang QZ, Miyamoto M, Furuichi Y, Komiyama T. (2006). Identification and characterization of a neutralizing monoclonal

antibody for the epitope on HM-1 killer toxin. *J. Biochem.*, 139, 399-406.

[48] Dziadek S, Jacques S, Bundle DR. (2008). A novel linker methodology for the synthesis of tailored conjugate vaccines composed of complex carbohydrate antigens and specific TH-cell peptide epitopes. *Chemistry*, 14, 5908-17.

[49] Vora S, Purimetla N, Brummer E, Stevens DA. (1998). Activity of voriconazole, a new triazole, combined with neutrophils on monocytes against *Candida albicans*: Effect of granulocyte colony-stimulating factor and granulocyte-monocyte colony stimulating factor. *Antimicrob. Agents Chemother.*, 42, 907-910.

[50] Ito JI, Lyons JM, Hong TB, Tamae D, Liu YK, Wilczynski SP, Kalkum M. (2006). Vaccinations with recombinant variants of *Aspergillus fumigatus* allergen Asp f 3 protect mice against invasive aspergillosis. *Infect. Immun.*, 74, 5075–5084.

[51] Selvakumar D, Miyamoto M, Furuichi Y, Komiyama T. (2006). Inhibition of fungal β-1,3-glucan synthase and cell growth by HM-1 killer toxin single-chain anti-idiotypic antibodies. *Antimicrob. Agents Chemother.*, 50, 3090–3097.

[52] Order SE, Stillwagon GB, Klein JL, Leichner PK, Siegelman SS, Fishman EK, Ettinger DS, Haulk T, Kopher K, Finney K. (1985). Iodine 131 antiferritin, a new treatment modality in hepatoma: a Radiation Therapy Oncology Group study. *J. Clin. Oncol.*, 3, 1573-1582.

[53] Dadachova E, Casadevall A. (2009). Radioimmunotherapy of Infectious Diseases. *Semin. Nucl. Med.*, 39, 146-153.

[54] Dadachova E, Casadevall A. (2006). Treatment of infection with radiolabeled antibodies. *Q. J. Nucl. Med. Mol. Imaging*, 50, 193-204.

[55] Dadachova E, Bryan RA, Huang X, Ortiz G, Moadel T, Casadevall A. (2007). Comparative evaluation of capsular polysaccharide-specific IgM and IgG antibodies and F(ab')2 and Fab fragments as delivery vehicles for radioimmunotherapy of fungal infection. *Clin. Cancer Res.*, 13, 5629s-5635s.

[56] Goldenberg DM, Sharkey RM, Udem S, Vagg R, Levine GM, Conte P, Swayne LC, Hansen HJ, Cunniff D, Anton J, Linke MJ, Smulian AG, Walzer PD. (1994). Immunoscintigraphy of *Pneumocystis carinii* pneumonia in AIDS patients. *J. Nucl. Med.*, 35, 1028-1034.

[57] Grieb TA, Forng RY, Stafford RE, Lin J, Almeida J, Bogdansky S, Ronholdt C, Drohan WN, Burgess WH. (2005). Effective use of

optimized, high-dose (50 kGy) gamma irradiation for pathogen inactivation of human bone allografts. *Biomaterials*, 26, 2033-2042.

[58] Dadachova E, Nakouzi A, Bryan R, Casadevall A. (2003). Ionizing radiation delivered by specific antibody is therapeutic against a fungal infection. *Proc. Natl. Acad. Sci. USA*, 100, 10942-10947.

[59] Dadachova E, Howell RW, Bryan RA, Frenkel A, Nosanchuk JD, Casadevall A. (2004). Susceptibility of human pathogens *Cryptococcus neoformans* and *Histoplasma capsulatum* to gamma radiation versus radioimmunotherapy with alpha- and beta emitting radioisotopes. *J. Nucl. Med.*, 45, 313-320.

[60] Martinez LR, Bryan RA, Apostolidis C, Morgenstern A, Casadevall A, Dadachova E. (2006). Antibody-guided alpharadiation effectively damages fungal biofilms. *Antimicrob. Agents Chemother.*, 50, 2132-2136.

[61] Dadachova E, Bryan RA, Frenkel A, Zhang T, Apostolidis C, Nosanchuk JS, Nosanchuk JD, Casadevall A. (2004). Evaluation of acute hematologic and long-term pulmonary toxicities of radioimmunotherapy of *Cryptococcus neoformans* infection in murine models. *Antimicrob. Agents Chemother.*, 48, 1004-1006.

[62] Bryan RA, Jiang Z, Huang X, Morgenstern A, Bruchertseifer F, Sellers R, Casadevall A, Dadachova E. (2009). Radioimmunotherapy is effective against high-inoculum *Cryptococcus neoformans* infection in mice and does not select for radiation-resistant cryptococcal cells. *Antimicrob. Agents Chemother.*, 53, 1679-1682.

[63] Dadachova E, Bryan RA, Apostolidis C, Morgenstern A, Zhang T, Moadel T, Torres M, Huang X, Revskaya E, Casadevall A. (2006). Interaction of radiolabeled antibodies with fungal cells and components of the immune system *in vitro* and during radioimmunotherapy for experimental fungal infection. *J. Infect. Dis.*, 193, 1427-1436.

[64] Zhou Q, Gault RA, Kozel TR, Murphy WJ. (2007). Protection from direct cerebral *Cryptococcus* infection by interferon-dependent activation of microglial cells. *J. Immunol.*, 178, 5753–5761.

[65] Nimrichter L, Barreto-Bergter E, Mendonca-Filho RR, Kneipp LF, Mazzi MT, Salve P, Farias SE, Wait R, Alviano CS, Rodrigues ML. (2004). A monoclonal antibody to glucosylceramide inhibits the growth of *Fonsecaea pedrosoi* and enhances the antifungal action of mouse macrophages. *Microbes Infect.*, 6, 657-665.

[66] Sutherland A, Ellis D. (2008). Treatment of a critically ill child with disseminated *Candida glabrata* with a recombinant human antibody

specific for fungal heat shock protein 90 and liposomal amphotericin B, caspofungin, and voriconazole. *Pediatr. Crit. Care Med.*, 9, e23-25.

[67] Kanu A, Patel K. (2008). Treatment of allergic bronchopulmonary aspergillosis (ABPA) in CF with anti-IgE antibody (omalizumab). *Pediatr. Pulmonol.*, 43, 1249-1251.

[68] de Jonge R, Thomma BP. (2009. Fungal LysM effectors: extinguishers of host immunity? *Trends Microbiol.*, 17(4), 151-157.

[69] Segal B, Leto T, Gallin J, Malech H, Holland S. (2000). Genetic, biochemical, and clinical features of chronic granulomatous disease. *Medicine (Baltimore)*, 79, 170–200.

[70] Tarcha EJ, Basrur V, Hung CY, Gardner MJ, Cole GT. (2006). Multivalent recombinant protein vaccine against coccidioidomycosis. *Infect. Immun.*, 74, 5802-5813.

[71] Larsen RA, Pappas PG, Perfect J, Aberg JA, Casadevall A, Cloud GA, James R, Filler S, Dismukes WE. (2005). Phase I evaluation of the safety and pharmacokinetics of murine-derived anticryptococcal antibody 18B7 in subjects with treated cryptococcal meningitis. *Antimicrob. Agents Chemother.*, 49, 952-958.

[72] Marques AF, da Silva MB, Juliano MA, Munhõz JE, Travassos LR, Taborda CP. (2008). Additive effect of P10 immunization and chemotherapy in anergic mice challenged intratracheally with virulent yeasts of *Paracoccidioides brasiliensis*. *Microbes Infect.*, 10, 1251-1258.

[73] Ibrahim AS, Spellberg BJ, Avenissian V, Fu Y, Filler SG, Edwards JE. (2005). Vaccination with recombinant N-terminal domain of Als1p improves survival during murine disseminated candidiasis by enhancing cell-mediated, not humoral, immunity. *Infect. Immun.*, 73, 999–1005.

[74] Spellberg B, Ibrahim AS, Yeaman MR, Lin L, Fu Y, Avanesian V, Bayer AS, Filler SG, Lipke P, Otoo H, Edwards JE Jr. (2008). The antifungal vaccine derived from the recombinant N terminus of Als3p protects mice against the bacterium *Staphylococcus aureus*. *Infect. Immun.*, 76, 4574-4580.

[75] Raska M, Belakova J, Wudattu NK, Kafková L, Růzicková K, Sebestová M, Kolár Z, Weigl E. (2005). Comparison of protective effect of protein and DNA vaccines hsp90 in murine model of systemic candidiasis. *Folia Microbiol.*, 50, 77-82.

[76] Gonzalez BE, Hulten KG, Lamberth L, Kaplan SL, Mason EO, the U.S. Pediatric Multicenter Pneumococcal Surveillance Group. (2006). *Streptococcus pneumoniae* serogroups 15 and 33: an increasing cause of pneumococcal infections in children in the United States after the

introduction of the pneumococcal 7-valent conjugate vaccine. *Pediatr. Infect. Dis. J.*, 25, 301–305.

[77] Hallander HO, Advani A, Donnelly D, Guftafsson L, Carlsson RM. (2005). Shifts of *Bordetella pertussis* variants in Sweden from 1970 to 2003 during the three periods marked by different vaccination programs. *J. Clin. Microbiol.*, 43, 2856–2865.

[78] Cowen LE, Lindquist S. (2005). Hsp90 potentiates the rapid evolution of new traits: drug resistance in diverse fungi. *Science*, 309, 2185-2189.

INDEX

A

B

C

D

H

I

J

K

L

M

N

V

W

X

Y

Z